PHOBIAS
REVEALED AND EXPLAINED

RICHARD WATERS

BARRON'S

First edition for the United States and Canada
published in 2004 by
Barron's Educational Series, Inc.

All inquiries should be addressed to:
Barron's Educational Series, Inc
250 Wireless Boulevard
Hauppauge, New York 11788
http://www.barronseduc.com

International Standard Book No. 0-7641-2667-9

Library of Congress Catalog Card No. 2003102258

Conceived, designed and produced by
Quid Publishing Ltd
Fourth Floor
Sheridan House
112-116a Western Road
Hove BN3 1DD
England
www.quidpublishing.com

Publisher: Nigel Browning
Design and Picture Research: Lindsey Johns
Editor: Leonie Taylor

Printed and Bound in China by Regent Publishing Services.

NOTE

PHOBIAS
REVEALED AND EXPLAINED

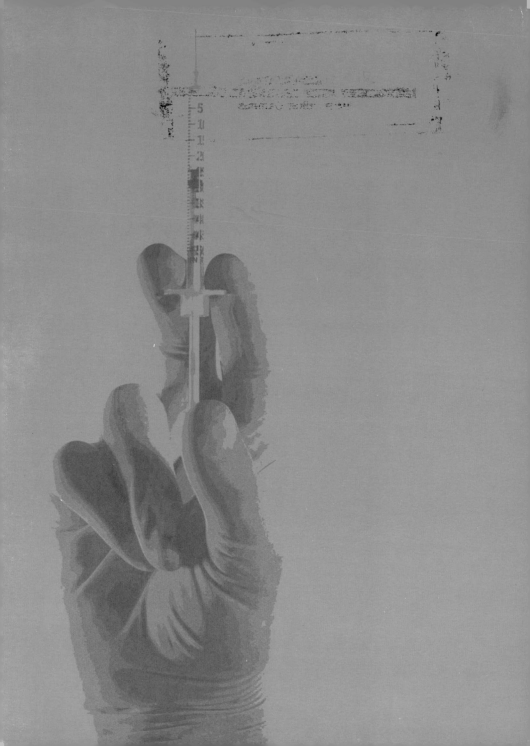

contents

foreword

Dramatic? Well, such are the acute symptoms of someone suffering an everyday phobia. I say "everyday," as according to The National Institute of Mental Health, between 5.1 and 12.5 percent of Americans have phobias. Furthermore, phobias are the most common psychiatric illness among women of all ages, and the second most common illness among men over the age of 25. They can develop anytime, anywhere and can happen to anyone. Nobody is immune and, as you'll see in this book, most of these terms that describe panic disorders have names that are rooted in Ancient Greek. In fact, the word "phobia" is Greek for "fear." Fear is an age-old phenomena, a yardstick for common sense and sometimes, when it becomes irrational, as in the case of many of the 100s of phobias collated here, a cross to bear.

While we've developed medical responses – drugs or psychotherapy – to combat this disorder, few can explain the origins of phobias. Indeed, a certain mystery remains – despite man's ability to send space probes into the corners of the solar system, we still can't fathom the darkness of our own minds.

Some phobias can be hereditary: a close friend of mine is Hemophobic (afraid of blood) and his son has inherited this terror. The merest mention of someone having an accident and bleeding can spiral both men into an anxiety attack that is closely followed by fainting. Once, when the father cut his finger in the kitchen and subsequently passed out, his son went to investigate – five minutes later, his wife found both father and son out cold on the kitchen floor.

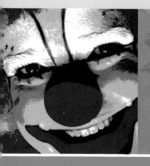
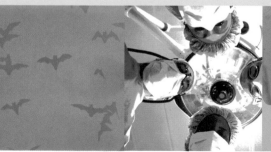
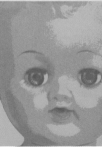

Some phobias pass away with time: for example, Nyctophobia (fear of darkness), which is often experienced by children. Others continue without rhyme or reason: an individual who effortlessly jumps out of airplanes may be unable to ride above the fourth floor on an elevator. I recently heard about a lady who had to conduct a job interview in the lobby of a tall building because the premises of the company she was applying to were on the sixteenth floor. The meeting was successful and she was offered the position, but she couldn't accept it because of her phobia.

Another friend used to drive an extra ten miles every day to avoid going through a tunnel on his way to work. Yes, he agreed, it cost him a considerable amount more in gas, but anything was better than the uncontrollable panic and rapid heartbeat that came on from the mere thought about driving through the tunnel. This is, perhaps, how we should define a phobia: a dread of something to such an extent that it interferes with our ability to work, socialize, and go about our daily routine.

This book has divided these many fears into accessible sections. It also sheds a little light on the etymology of the phobias, that is to say, how their meaning was formed.

What struck me in the writing and research of this project was twofold. First, what would we do without our Greek predecessors? That their language and beliefs survived, were adopted and renamed by the Romans, to endure to the present day in our own modern tongue is a testament to their intelligence and imagination. Second, but perhaps more importantly, it strikes me that two-and-a-half millennia later, we are still prone to exactly the same fears, with some new paranoias added in response to modern living.

As you'll know from your own deepest fears, they can be irrational, unsettling, and maddening, but they are ultimately, essential components of who we are.

Richard Waters

MOON

SELENOPHOBIA
Se-lay-no-foe-bee-ah
Often related to
superstitions of what
may befall on a full
moon, this term
originates directly from
the Greek word *seleno*,
meaning the moon.

Related Phobias:
HELIOPHOBIA, fear of the sun

CELESTIAL SPACES

ASTROPHOBIA
Ast-row-foe-bee-ah
Astra is the Greek word for
star, giving us the origin of
this term which describes
individuals who fear their
destiny being ruled by the
stars and planets.

METEORS

METEOROPHOBIA
Me-tee-oro-foe-bee-ah
As with cometophobia,
the meaning of this term can
be traced to the Greek word
meteoro, meaning lofty
or heavenly body.

Related Phobias:
ATEPHOBIA, fear of disasters

COMETS

COMETOPHOBIA
Com-it-oh-foe-bee-ah
The word *comet* is a
modern derivation of the
Greek *meteoro*, which
means lofty or raised up
in the air (i.e. the planets).
Thus, Cometophobia is the
dread of meteors and comets.

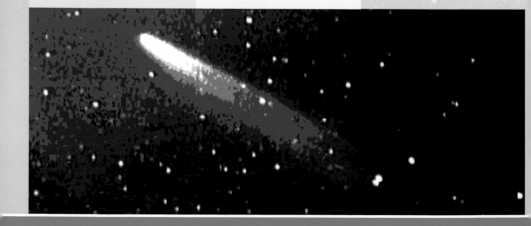

STARS

SIDEROPHOBIA
Si-der-o-foe-bee-ah
This excessive fear that something evil might arise due to the influence of the stars, finds its origin in the Latin word *sidero*, meaning star.

Related Phobias:
MYTHOPHOBIA, fear of myths

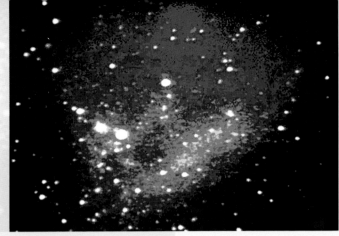

OUTER SPACE

SPACEPHOBIA
Sp-ey-si-foe-bee-ah
The modern words space and spacious are derivations of the Latin suffix *acious*, meaning abounding in. In the case of this phobia, it literally translates as *fear of vastness*.

Related Phobias:
APEIROPHOBIA, fear of infinity

COSMIC PHENOMENON

KOSMIKOPHOBIA
Cos-mik-oh-foe-bee-ah
This term emanates from the Greek word *cosmo*, meaning the universe.

NORTHERN LIGHTS

AURORAPHOBIA
Or-ora-foe-bee-ah
This unusual fear of the luminous Aurora Borealis derives from the Latin word *aurora* meaning dawn.

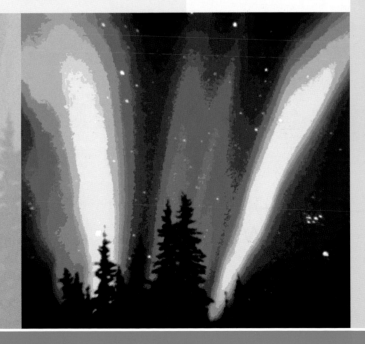

BIRDS

ORNITHOPHOBIA
Or-nith-o-foe-bee-ah
The Greek for bird – *ornitho* –
gives direct meaning to this
phobia of feathered things.

Related Phobias:
AEROPHOBIA, fear of flying

FEATHERS OR BEING TICKLED BY FEATHERS

PTERONOPHOBIA
Tear-o-no-foe-bee-ah
This phobia finds its
derivation in the Greek
word *ptero*, meaning winged
or feather-like.

SHARKS

SELACHOPHOBIA
Say-lak-o-foe-bee-ah
or
GALEPHOBIA
Gal-ay-foe-bee-ah
No direct Greek or Latin
word can be found to
explain this logical phobia.
However, the known Greek
word for shark is *galeo*.

Related Phobias:
ODONTOPHOBIA, fear of teeth,
especially animal

SHELLFISH

OSTRACONOPHOBIA
Os-tra-con-o-foe-bee-ah
This abhorrence of mollusks finds its origin in the Greek word *ostracon*, meaning shell or oyster.

Related Phobias:
EMETOPHOBIA, fear of vomiting

CHICKENS

ALEKTOROPHOBIA
A-lek-tor-o-foe-bee-ah
Fear of chickens finds its meaning in the Greek word for rooster – *alektor*. While it relates to the birds themselves, alive or dead, this phobia may also include a fear of their eggs.

FISH

ICHTHYOPHOBIA
Itch-thy-o-foe-bee-ah
Ichthyois, the Greek word for fish, explains the derivation of this aquatic phobia.

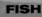

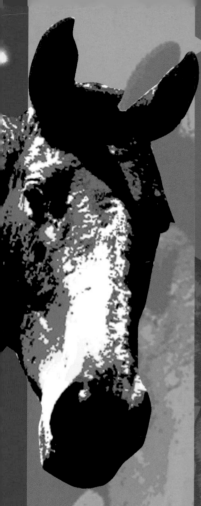

CATS

ACLUROPHOBIA
Ac-lur-o-foe-bee-ah
or
AILUROPHOBIA
Ay-lur-o-foe-bee-ah
or
ELUROPHOBIA
El-ur-o-foe-bee-ah
or
FELINOPHOBIA
Fee-line-o-foe-bee-ah
or
GALEOPHOBIA
Ga-ley-o-foe-bia
or
GATOPHOBIA
Gay-to-foe-bee-ah
Acturo, alluro, and *eluro* are all variants of the Greek word for cat. Felinophobia, galephobia (see also sharks), and gatophobia represent exactly the same dread of cats yet are derived from the Latin words, *feli, galeo,* and *gato.*

Related Phobias:
WICCAPHOBIA, fear of witchcraft

DOGS

CYNOPHOPBIA
SY-NO-FOE-BEE-AH
The Greek word for dog is *cyno,* and so Cynophobia is canine-inspired terror.

Related Phobias:
AMYCHOPHOBIA, fear of being scratched by puppies, dogs, kittens, or cats

ANIMALS

ZOOPHOBIA
Zu-foe-bee-ah
The Greek word for animal is *zoo.* Phobics of this disorder can be scared by both the attention and the presence of animals.

FUR OR ANIMAL SKIN

DORAPHOBIA
Door-ah-foe-bee-ah
Dora is the Greek word for hide or skin. Doraphobia is, therefore, the morbid fear of touching animal skin or fur.

Related Phobias:
TEXTOPHOBIA, fear of touching certain fabrics.

HORSES

EQUINOPHOBIA
Eq-wine-o-foe-bee-ah
or
HIPPOPHOBIA
Hip-po-foe-bee-ah
Equus is the Latin and *hippo* the Greek for horse, giving name to this abject fear of horses.

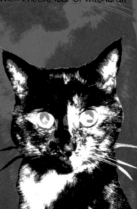

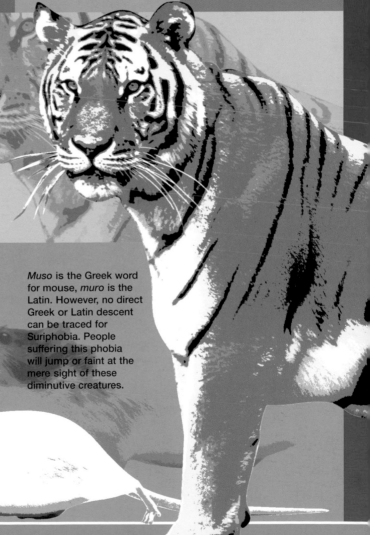

BULLS

TAURAPHOBIA
Tor-o-foe-bee-ah
Tauro is the Greek word
for bull. As far back as
the ancient Minoan culture,
these creatures were
worshipped and revered,
but not by tauraphobics.

RATS, MOLES

ZEMMIPHOBIA
Zem-my-foe-bee-ah
No direct word, Latin or
Greek, can be found to
explain the origin of this fear.

OTTERS

LUTRAPHOBIA
Lew-tra-foe-bee-ah
The origins for this phobia are
found in the Latin word *lutra*,
relating to otters or furry,
aquatic animals.

WILD ANIMALS

AGRIZOOPHOBIA
Ag-ree-zoo-foe-bee-ah
The Greek word for animals is
zoo. Add to this the Latin
word *agri*, meaning savage,
and it is easy to see where
this phobia of wild animals
finds its origin.

Related Phobias:
HYDROPHOBOPHOBIA, fear of
catching rabies

MICE

MUSOPHOBIA
Mew-so-foe-bee-ah
or
MUROPHOBIA
Mure-o-foe-bee-ah
or
SURIPHOBIA
Sur-I-foe-bee-ah

Muso is the Greek word
for mouse, *muro* is the
Latin. However, no direct
Greek or Latin descent
can be traced for
Suriphobia. People
suffering this phobia
will jump or faint at the
mere sight of these
diminutive creatures.

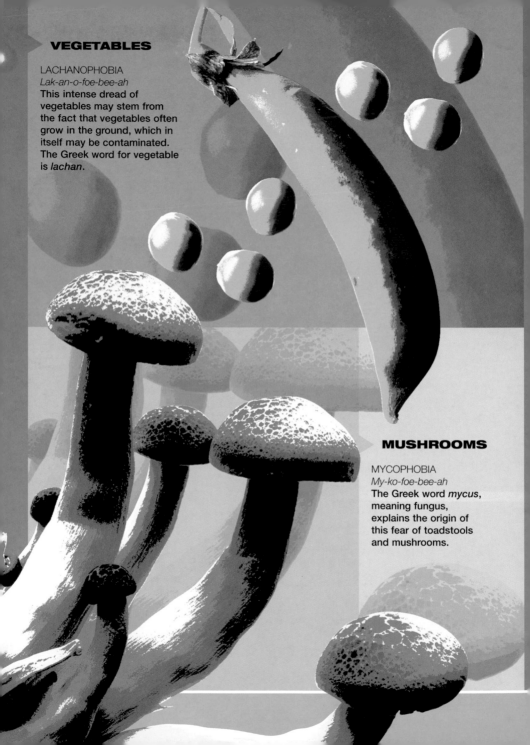

VEGETABLES

LACHANOPHOBIA
Lak-an-o-foe-bee-ah
This intense dread of
vegetables may stem from
the fact that vegetables often
grow in the ground, which in
itself may be contaminated.
The Greek word for vegetable
is *lachan*.

MUSHROOMS

MYCOPHOBIA
My-ko-foe-bee-ah
The Greek word *mycus*,
meaning fungus,
explains the origin of
this fear of toadstools
and mushrooms.

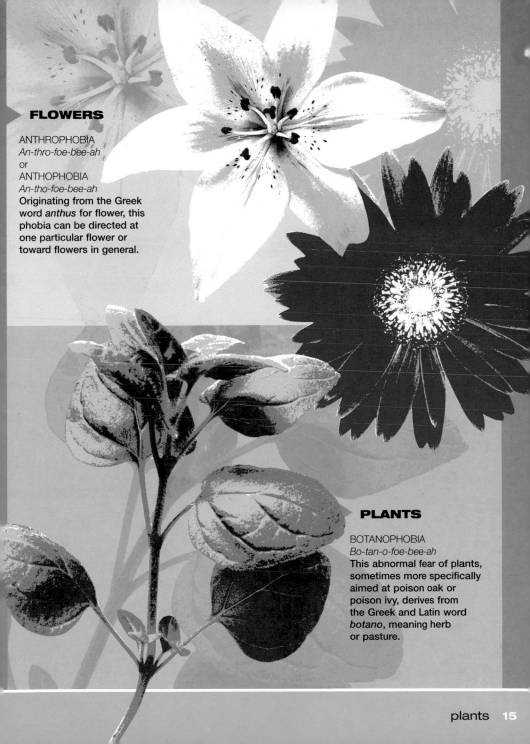

FLOWERS

ANTHROPHOBIA
An-thro-foe-bee-ah
or
ANTHOPHOBIA
An-tho-foe-bee-ah
**Originating from the Greek
word *anthus* for flower, this
phobia can be directed at
one particular flower or
toward flowers in general.**

PLANTS

BOTANOPHOBIA
Bo-tan-o-foe-bee-ah
**This abnormal fear of plants,
sometimes more specifically
aimed at poison oak or
poison ivy, derives from
the Greek and Latin word
botano, meaning herb
or pasture.**

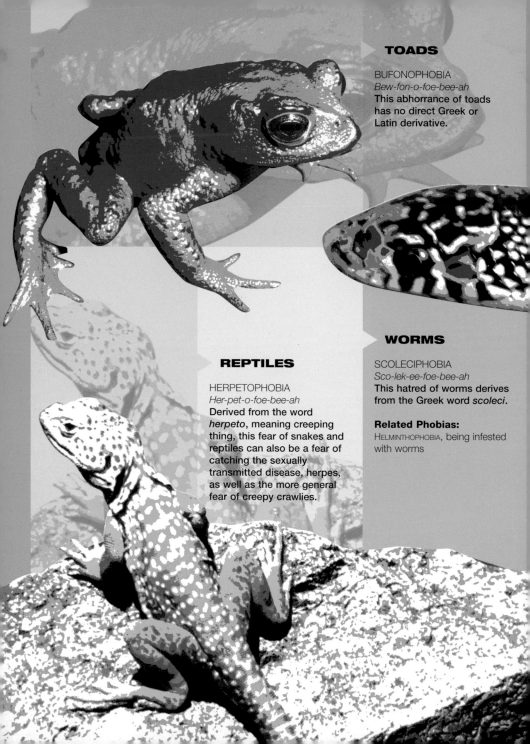

TOADS

BUFONOPHOBIA
Bew-fon-o-foe-bee-ah
This abhorrance of toads
has no direct Greek or
Latin derivative.

WORMS

SCOLECIPHOBIA
Sco-lek-ee-foe-bee-ah
This hatred of worms derives
from the Greek word *scoleci*.

Related Phobias:
HELMINTHOPHOBIA, being infested
with worms

REPTILES

HERPETOPHOBIA
Her-pet-o-foe-bee-ah
Derived from the word
herpeto, meaning creeping
thing, this fear of snakes and
reptiles can also be a fear of
catching the sexually
transmitted disease, herpes,
as well as the more general
fear of creepy crawlies.

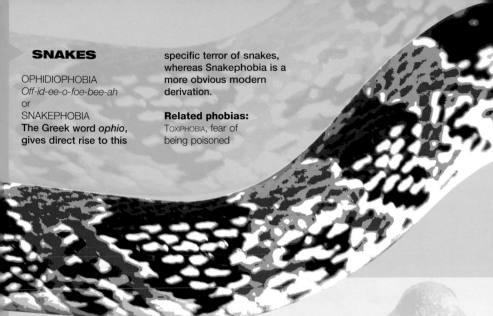

SNAKES

OPHIDIOPHOBIA
Off-id-ee-o-foe-bee-ah
or
SNAKEPHOBIA
The Greek word *ophio*,
gives direct rise to this specific terror of snakes,
whereas Snakephobia is a
more obvious modern
derivation.

Related phobias:
TOXIPHOBIA, fear of
being poisoned

TAPEWORMS

TAENIOPHOBIA
Tay-nee-o-foe-bee-ah
This excessive fear of
tapeworms, and the personal
physical damage they can
inflict, emanates from the
Greek word *taenio*, meaning
ribbon or band.

Related Phobias:
PARASITOPHOBIA, fear of parasites

FROGS

BATRACHOPHOBIA
Bat-rak-o-foe-bee-ah
An aversion to frogs,
newts, toads, and slimy
things, this phobia finds its
root in the Greek word for
frog – *batrach*.

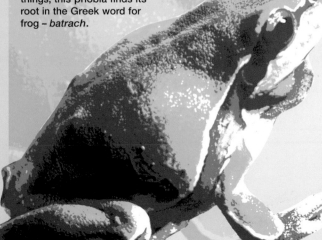

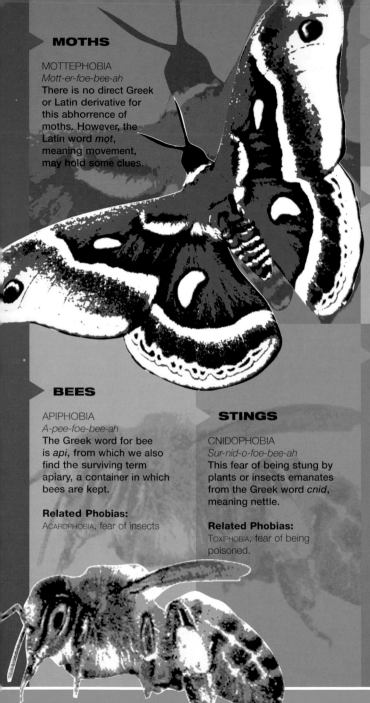

MOTHS

MOTTEPHOBIA
Mott-er-foe-bee-ah
There is no direct Greek or Latin derivative for this abhorrence of moths. However, the Latin word *mot*, meaning movement, may hold some clues.

PARASITES

PARASITOPHOBIA
Para-sit-o-foe-bee-ah
This dread of parasites finds its root in the Greek verb *parasito*, which means to eat beside.

WASPS

SPHEKSOPHOBIA
Sfek-so-foe-bee-ah
This uncontrollable fear of wasps directly originates from the Greek word *spheco*, meaning wasp.

INSECTS

ACAROPHOBIA
Ak-aro-foe-bee-ah
or
ENTOMOPHOBIA
En-toe-mo-foe-bee-ah
or
INSECTOMOPHOBIA
Acar is Greek for mite or tick, while the Greek word *entom* literally means in pieces, like the segmented form of a millipede. Sufferers of actaphobia specifically fear insects that cause itching. There is no Greek or Latin derivative for insectophobia.

Related Phobias:
Microphobia, fear of small things

BEES

APIPHOBIA
A-pee-foe-bee-ah
The Greek word for bee is *api*, from which we also find the surviving term apiary, a container in which bees are kept.

Related Phobias:
Acarophobia, fear of insects

STINGS

CNIDOPHOBIA
Sur-nid-o-foe-bee-ah
This fear of being stung by plants or insects emanates from the Greek word *cnid*, meaning nettle.

Related Phobias:
Toxiphobia, fear of being poisoned.

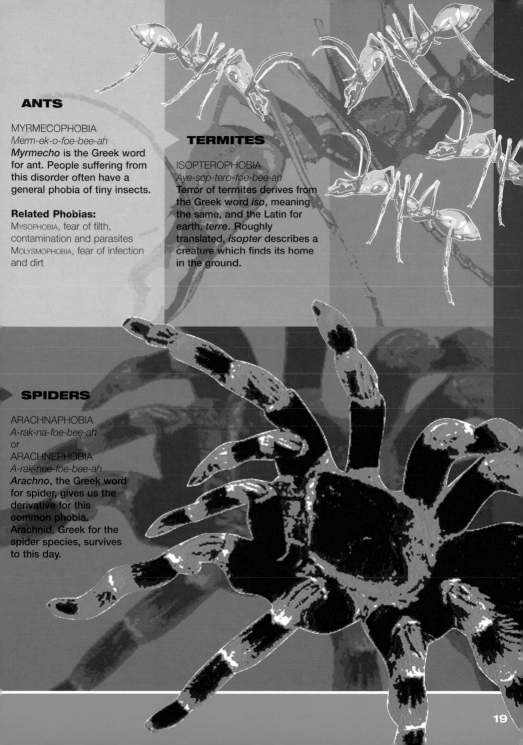

ANTS

MYRMECOPHOBIA
Merm-ek-o-foe-bee-ah
Myrmecho is the Greek word
for ant. People suffering from
this disorder often have a
general phobia of tiny insects.

Related Phobias:
MYSOPHOBIA, fear of filth,
contamination and parasites
MOLYSMOPHOBIA, fear of infection
and dirt

TERMITES

ISOPTEROPHOBIA
Aye-sop-tero-foe-bee-ah
Terror of termites derives from
the Greek word *iso*, meaning
the same, and the Latin for
earth, *terre*. Roughly
translated, *isopter* describes a
creature which finds its home
in the ground.

SPIDERS

ARACHNAPHOBIA
A-rak-na-foe-bee-ah
or
ARACHNEPHOBIA
A-rak-nee-foe-bee-ah
Arachno, the Greek word
for spider, gives us the
derivative for this
common phobia.
Arachnid, Greek for the
spider species, survives
to this day.

WATER

HYDROPHOBIA
Hi-dro-foe-bee-ah
This fear derives in meaning from the Greek word *hydro*, meaning water. The same word also begets such modern usages as rehydrate, hydrofoil and hydrant.

Related Phobias:
ABLUTOPHOBIA, fear of washing

SEA OR OCEAN

THALASSOPHOBIA
Tha-lass-oh-foe-bee-ah
This fear of the sea or huge bodies of water is derived from the Greek word *thalasso*, meaning sea.

Related Phobias:
CENOPHOBIA, fear of empty places

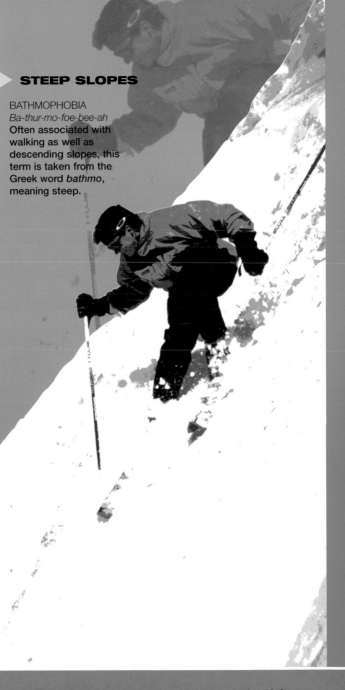

CAVES

TROGLOPHOBIA
Tr-og-lo-foe-bee-ah
Troglo is the Greek word for cave dweller, from which we also derive the anthropological term troglodyte.

STEEP SLOPES

BATHMOPHOBIA
Ba-thur-mo-foe-bee-ah
Often associated with walking as well as descending slopes, this term is taken from the Greek word *bathmo*, meaning steep.

FLOODS

ANTLOPHOBIA
Ant-lo-foe-bee-ah
There are no Greek or Latin words that can explain the origins of this term.

Related Phobias:
HYDROPHOBIA, fear of water

LAKES

LIMNOPHOBIA
Lim-no-foe-bee-ah
An extreme fear, Limnophobia finds its origin in the Greek word *limno*, meaning marsh, lake, or pool.

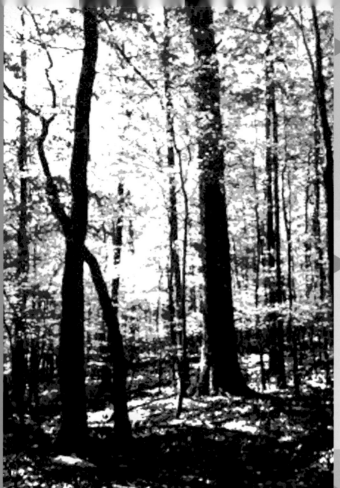

WOODS AT NIGHT

NYCTOHYLOPHOBIA
Nik-toe-hi-lo-foe-bee-ah
Nycto and *hylo* are the Greek words for night and wood; literally combined, they describe a fear of woods at night.

FORESTS OR WOODEN OBJECTS

XYLOPHOBIA
Zy-lo-foe-bee-ah
This excessive fear of wooden objects or indeed woods, finds its origin in the Greek word for wood – *xylo*.

Related Phobias:
DENDROPHOBIA, fear of trees.

TREES

DENDROPHOBIA
Den-dro-foe-bee-ah
Dendro is the Greek word for tree, which provides us with a clear explanation of this term's evolution.

FORESTS

HYLOPHOBIA
Hi-lo-foe-bee-ah
Sometimes referring to a fear of woods but also a hatred of materialism, this term is derived from the Greek word *hylo*, meaning forest.

Related Phobias:
LYGOPHOBIA, fear of dark or gloomy places

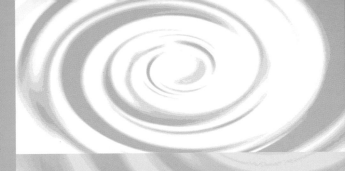

RIVERS

POTAMPHOBIA
Pot-am-foe-bee-ah
or
POTAMOPHOBIA
Pot-am-o-foe-bee-ah
Potamo is the Greek word for river, explaining the source of this fear of rivers and running water.

WHIRLPOOLS

DINOPHOBIA
Dye-no-foe-bee-ah
This unsettling anxiety derives in meaning from the Greek word *dino*, meaning whirling or full of eddies.

WAVES OR WAVE-LIKE MOTIONS

KYMOPHOBIA
Ky-mo-foe-bee-ah
or
CYMOPHOBIA
Si-mo-foe-bee-ah

The Greek word for wave, *kymo*, gives us the origin of this fear. Sufferers of this disorder can, as well as having a fear of the motion of waves, also be afraid of rolling undulations in the landscape.

Related Phobias:
KINESSOPHOBIA, fear of motion

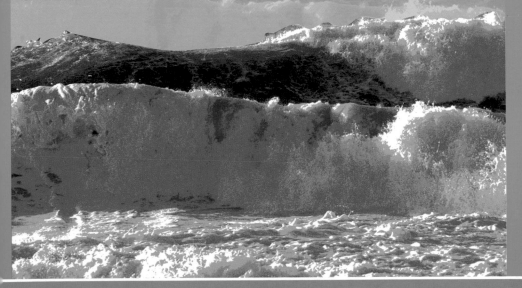

DARKNESS

ACHLUOPHOBIA
Ash-lu-o-foe-bee-ah
or
SCOPTOPHOBIA
Sk-op-toe-foe-bee-ah
Achlyo and ***skoto*** are both Greek for darkness. Both phobias relate to an abject dread of darkness.

CLOUDS

NEPHOPHOBIA
Ne-fo-foe-bee-ah
Nephelo is the Greek word for clouds, explaining the origins of this term.

Related Phobias:
URANOPHOBIA, fear of heaven

NIGHT

NOCTIPHOBIA
Nok-ti-foe-bee-ah
or
NYCTOPHOBIA
Nyk-toe-foe-bee-ah

These twin phobias derive from the Latin word *nocti* and the Greek equivalent *nycto* meaning the night. Sufferers often fear what calamities and doom the night may bring.

Related Phobias:
PHASMOPHOBIA, fear of ghosts
ACHLUOPHOBIA, fear of darkness

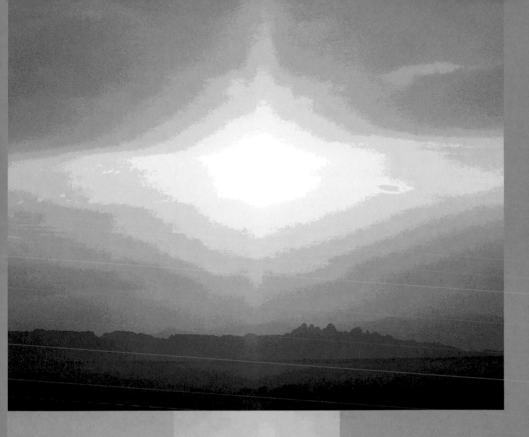

SUN OR SUNLIGHT

HELIOPHOBIA
He-lee-o-foe-bee-ah
This aversion to sunlight originates in meaning from the Greek word *helio*, meaning sun. Phobics of this disorder often fear contracting skin cancer from exposure.

Related Phobias:
DERMATOSIOPHOBIA, fear of skin disease

DAWN OR DAYLIGHT

EOSOPHOBIA
Ee-oss-o-foe-bee-ah
This hatred of the dawn can be traced to the Greek word *eoso*, meaning daybreak or dawn. Sufferers sometimes dread the approach of a new day because they may be seen by others.

Related Phobias:
SCOPTOPHOBIA, fear of being looked at

DAYLIGHT OR SUNSHINE

PHENGOPHOBIA
Fen-go-foe-bee-ah
An excessive fear of daylight, this term finds its origin in the Greek word *phengo*, meaning splendor, luster, or daylight.

Related Phobias:
CHEROPHOBIA, fear of gaiety

AIR

ANEMOPHOBIA
A-ne-mo-foe-bee-ah

This phobia holds sufferers in fear not only of wind, but also of approaching storms and sometimes even mere drafts. The origin of this term can be traced to the Greek word *anemo*, meaning wind or breath.

Related Phobias:

AERONAUSIPHOBIA, fear of air sickness

FOG

HOMICHLOPHOBIA
Hom-ich-lo-foe-bee-ah
or
NEBULAPHOBIA
Neb-you-la-foe-bee-ah

Although there are no Latin or Greek words to illuminate the origin of Homichlophobia, Nebulaphobia clearly emanates from the Latin word *nebula*, meaning fog.

Related Phobias:

SPECTROPHOBIA, fear of specters

COLD

CHEIMAPHOBIA
Chay-ma-foe-bee-ah
or
PSYCHROPHOBIA
Sy-cro-foe-bee-ah
or
FRIGOPHOBIA
Fri-joe-foe-bee-ah

The Greek words *psychro*, meaning cold, and *cheimo*, meaning winter, illuminate the origins of these terms. The Latin *frigo*, from which we derive modern words such as refrigerate, means cold.

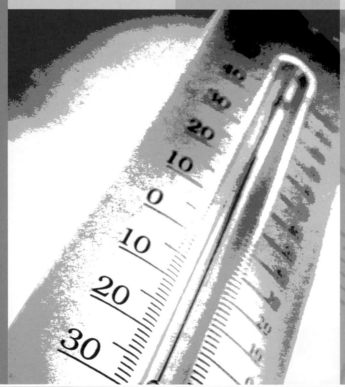

HEAT

THERMOPHOBIA
Th-ur-mo-foe-bee-ah

This loathing of heat or humidity takes its name from the Greek word *thermo*, meaning heat or hot. Modern derivations, to name but a few, include: thermostat, thermos flask, and thermometer.

ICE OR FROST

PAGOPHBOIA
Paj-o-foe-bee-ah
Pago is the Greek word for ice or frost, providing us with a clear origin of this aversion to ice.

Related Phobias:
DYSTYCHIPHOBIA, fear of accidents

EXTREME COLD

CRYOPHOBIA
Cry-o-foe-bee-ah
This excessive fear of ice and cold emanates from the Greek word *cryo*, meaning frost or ice. Once again, the Greek word has survived in the modern western tongue in terms such as cryogenics – the freezing of dead bodies for rejuvenation later.

WIND

ANCRAOPHOBIA
An-cre-o-foe-bee-ah
or
ANEMOPHOBIA
A-ne-mo-foe-bee-ah
The origins of ancraophobia are obscure and cannot be traced in either Latin or Greek. *Anemo*, however, is the Greek word for wind, explaining the root of Anemophobia.

Related Phobias:
KINESSOPHOBIA, fear of motion

THUNDER AND LIGHTNING

ASTRAPHOBIA
Ass-tra-foe-bee-ah
or
KERAUNOPHOBIA
Ke-raw-no-foe-bee-ah
The Greek words *astra*,
meaning star or of the
heavens, and *cerauno*,
meaning thunderbolt or
crusher provide us with the
roots of these terms.

Related Phobias:
ELECTROPHOBIA, fear of electricity

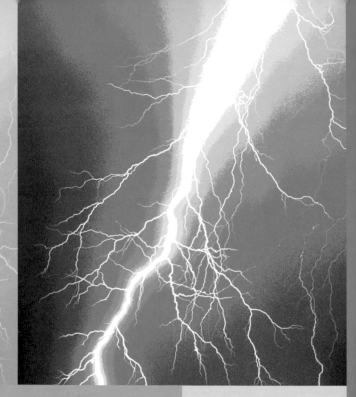

RAIN

OMBROPHOBIA
Om-bro-foe-bee-ah
or
PLUVIOPHOBIA
Pl-oo-vee-o-foe-bee-ah
Ombro is Greek for rain and
pluvio is Latin. Both describe
an excessive anxiety over
rain.

Related Phobias:
HYDROPHOBIA, fear of water

MOISTURE, DAMPNESS OR LIQUIDS

HYGROPHOBIA
Hi-grow-foe-bee-ah
This aversion to moisture and
sometimes water and wine
emanates from the Greek word
hygro, meaning moist.

Related Phobias:
XEROPHOBIA, fear of dryness
or dry places

THUNDER STORMS

BRONTOPHOBIA
Br-on-toe-foe-bee-ah
Bronto is the Greek word for thunder and provides us with an easy explanation of this phobias heritage.

TORNADOES AND HURRICANES

LILAPSOPHOBIA
Li-lap-so-foe-bee-ah
This justified dread of tornadoes and hurricanes cannot be directly traced to any Greek or Latin word.

Related Phobias:
ATEPHOBIA, fear of catastrophe

SNOW

CHIONOPHOBIA
Chae-on-o-foe-bee-ah
This excessive fear of snow finds its origin in the Greek word for snow – *chion*.

Related Phobias:
LEUKOPHOBIA, fear of white

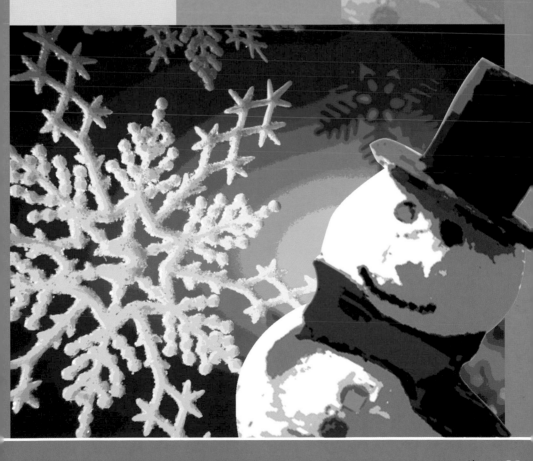

GOLD

AUROPHOBIA
Or-oh-foe-bee-ah
Sometimes referring to a fear of shiny things or emblems of wealth, aurophobia is directly descended from the Latin word *auro*, meaning gold.

Related Phobias:
CHROMETOPHOBIA, fear of money

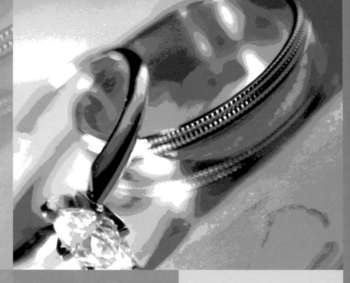

POISON

IOPHOBIA
Eye-o-foe-bee-ah
The origin of this term can be found in the Greek word *io*, meaning rust or poison.

Related Phobias:
TOXIPHOBIA, fear of being poisoned

GRAVITY

BAROPHOBIA
Ba-row-foe-bee-ah
This fear of heaviness or changes in air pressure originates from the Greek word *baro*, meaning heavy.

Related Phobias:
AEROPHOBIA, fear of drafts and air

DRAFTS

AEROPHOBIA
Air-oh-foe-bee-ah
or
ANEMOPHOBIA
A-nem-oh-foe-bee-ah
These debilitating fears find their direct word origins in the Greek words *aero*, meaning air, and *anemo*, meaning breath.

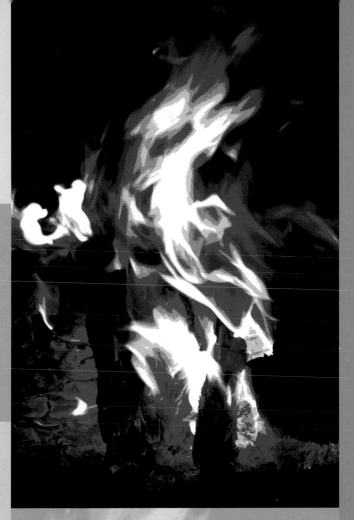

DECAYING MATTER

SEPLOPHOBIA
Sep-lo-foe-bee-ah
This term can be traced to the Greek word *septi*, meaning rot or decay. From this, we also arrive at such words as antiseptic or septicemia.

DUST

AMATHOPHOBIA
A-ma-tho-foe-bee-ah
or
KONIPHOBIA
Ko-nee-foe-bee-ah
These phobias of ingesting or being covered in dust emanate from the Greek words *amatho* and *koni*, both meaning sand or dust.

COMPLEX SCIENTIFIC TERMINOLOGY

HELLENOLOGOPHOBIA
Hel-len-ol-og-oh-foe-bee-ah
This fear of overly complex terminology also refers to a hatred of Greek words, as it is derives from *hellene*, the original word for the Greek language. It is unlikely that a hellenologophobic would like this term or be reading this book!

FIRE

ARSONPHOBIA
Ah-sun-foe-bee-ah
or
PYROPHOBIA
Py-row-foe-bee-ah
These excessive fears of being near or starting a fire can be traced to the Latin word *ars* and the Greek *pyro*, meaning fire.

Related Phobias:
THERMOPHOBIA, fear of heat

MICROBES

BACILLOPHOBIA
Ba-sil-o-foe-bee-ah
or
MICROBIOPHOBIA
My-cro-bio-foe-bee-ah
Bacillophobia derives from the Latin word *bacilli*, meaning rod-shaped, as in rod-shaped bacteria. Microbiophobia stems from the Greek words *micro*, meaning small, and *bio*, meaning life. Literally compounded, they translate as a fear of microscopic life-forms.

Related Phobias:
Pediculophobia, fear of lice

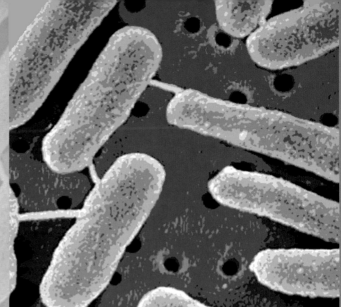

BACTERIA

BACTERIOPHOBIA
Bak-te-ree-o-foe-bee-ah
The origin of this word can be found in the Greek *bacterio*, meaning micro-organism. Sufferers of this dread often have a fear of not being sufficiently clean and therefore feel compelled to keep washing.

Related Phobias:
Automysophobia, fear of being dirty

GERMS

VERMINOPHOBIA
Vur-min-o-foe-bee-ah
Often relating to a fear of worms, this term is derived from the Latin word *vermo*, meaning worm.

Related Phobias:
Helminthophobia, fear of being infested by worms

FILTH OR DIRT

RHYPOPHOBIA
Rye-po-foe-bee-ah
or
RUPOPHOBIA
Ru-po-foe-bee-ah
This phobia originates in meaning from the Greek word *rhypo*, meaning filth.

CONTAMINATION FROM GERMS OR DIRT

MYSOPHOBIA
My-so-foe-bee-ah
or
MISOPHOBIA
Me-so-foe-bee-ah
This fear of uncleanliness derives from the Greek word *myso*, meaning dirt.

Related Phobias:
Coprophobia, fear of personal filth

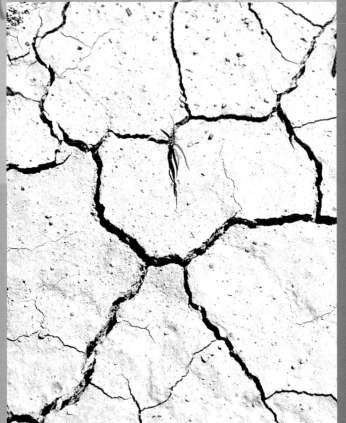

ELECTRICITY

ELECTROPHOBIA
Eh-lek-tro-foe-bee-ah
This term can be traced to the Latin word *electro*, meaning amber. In 1600, Dr. William Gilbert used the word to describe the action of producing static electricity by vigorously rubbing amber.

DRYNESS

XEROPHOBIA
Ze-row-foe-bee-ah
This aversion to dryness, often relating to deserts or arid places, finds its root in the Greek word *xero*, meaning dry.

INFECTION, CONTAMINATION OR DIRT

MOLYSMOPHOBIA
Mol-iss-mo-foe-bee-ah
or
MOLYSOMOPHOBIA
Mol-iss-o-mo-foe-bee-ah
This particular dread originates from the Greek word *molysmo*, meaning infection.

Related Phobias:
MYSOPHOBIA, fear of uncleanness

SMELL OR ODORS

OLFACTOPHOBIA
Ol-fak-toe-foe-bee-ah
This excessive fear of certain smells is derived in meaning from the Latin verb *olfacto*, meaning to smell.

Related Phobias:
GEUMAPHOBIA, fear of certain tastes

SLIME

BLENNOPHOBIA
Ble-no-foe-bee-ah
or
MYXOPHOBIA
Mix-o-foe-bee-ah
These identical fears find their origins in the Latin and Greek words *blenno* and *myxo*, both meaning mucus or slime.

Related Phobias:
TEXTOPHOBIA, fear of certain textures

BEING IN DARK PLACES

LYGOPHOBIA
Lie-go-foe-bee-ah
The Greek word *lygo* means shadow or darkness, which explains the root of this term.

Related Phobias:
NYCTOPHOBIA, fear of darkness

FLASHING LIGHT

SELAPHOBIA
Cel-a-foe-bee-ah
There are no Greek or Latin words that can sufficiently explain this terms origins.

Related Phobias:
AURORAPHOBIA, fear of the Northern Lights

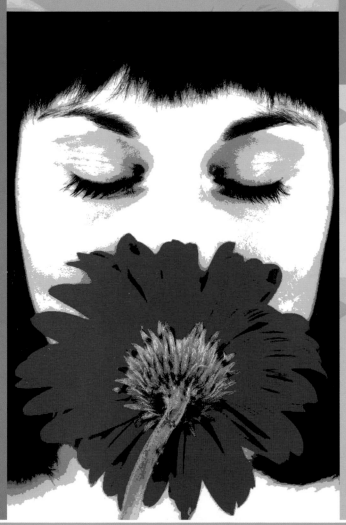

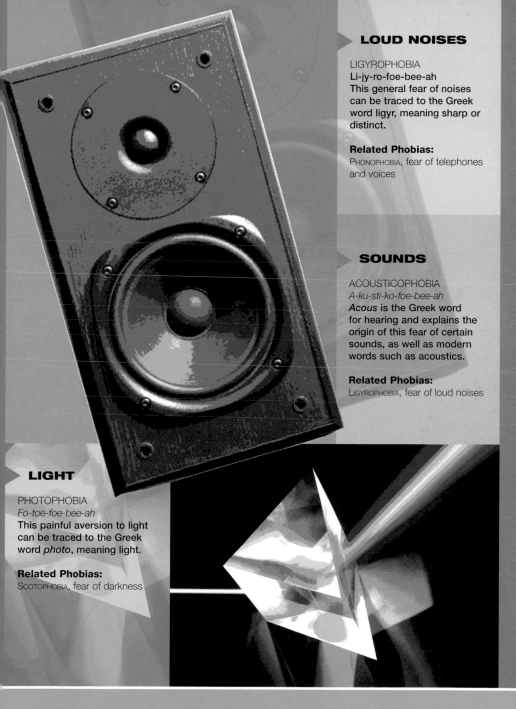

LOUD NOISES

LIGYROPHOBIA
Li-jy-ro-foe-bee-ah
This general fear of noises can be traced to the Greek word ligyr, meaning sharp or distinct.

Related Phobias:
PHONOPHOBIA, fear of telephones and voices

SOUNDS

ACOUSTICOPHOBIA
A-ku-sti-ko-foe-bee-ah
Acous is the Greek word for hearing and explains the origin of this fear of certain sounds, as well as modern words such as acoustics.

Related Phobias:
LIGYROPHOBIA, fear of loud noises

LIGHT

PHOTOPHOBIA
Fo-toe-foe-bee-ah
This painful aversion to light can be traced to the Greek word *photo*, meaning light.

Related Phobias:
SCOTOPHOBIA, fear of darkness

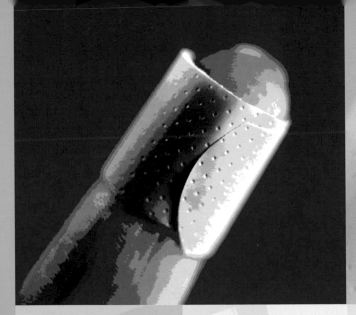

ACCIDENTS

DYSTYCHIPHOBIA
Dis-tae-chi-foe-bee-ah
This fear of risk-taking and personal injury finds its root in the Greek words *dys*, meaning bad or harsh, and *tycho*, meaning luck or fortune. Together, they combine to make ill-fortune.

Related Phobias:
TACHOPHOBIA, fear of speed

LEARNING

SOPHOPHOBIA
Sof-oh-foe-bee-ah
This hatred of learning derives in meaning from the Greek word *sopho*, meaning wise. Another contemporary derivation is the word *sophism*, meaning a false argument.

Related Phobias:
GNOSIOPHOBIA, fear of knowledge

SCHOOL

SCOLIONOPHOBIA
Sko-lee-oh-no-foe-bee-ah
There is no Greek or Latin word to explain the word origin of this global aversion to school.

TAKING TESTS

TESTOPHOBIA
Te-sto-foe-bee-ah
There is no Greek or Latin word that can explain the origin of this term but it is most likely a derivation of the modern word, test.

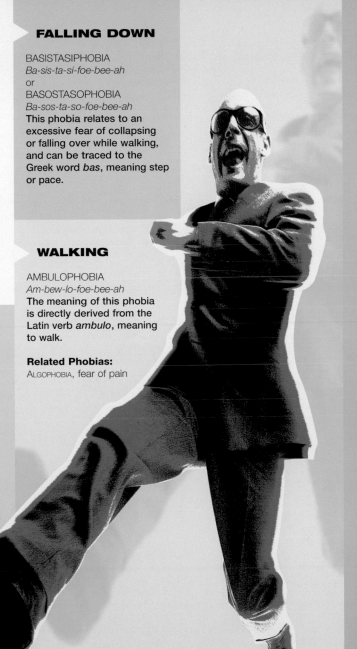

SOCIETY OR PEOPLE IN GENERAL

SOCIOPHOBIA
So-she-oh-foe-bee-ah
or
ANTHROPOPHOBIA
An-thro-poe-foe-bee-ah
This hatred of mixing with others derives from the Latin word for friendship – *socio* – while Anthropophobia emanates in meaning from the Greek word *anthropo*, meaning mankind.

FALLING DOWN

BASISTASIPHOBIA
Ba-sis-ta-si-foe-bee-ah
or
BASOSTASOPHOBIA
Ba-sos-ta-so-foe-bee-ah
This phobia relates to an excessive fear of collapsing or falling over while walking, and can be traced to the Greek word *bas*, meaning step or pace.

WALKING

AMBULOPHOBIA
Am-bew-lo-foe-bee-ah
The meaning of this phobia is directly derived from the Latin verb *ambulo*, meaning to walk.

Related Phobias:
ALGOPHOBIA, fear of pain

SCHOOL GOING TO

DIDASKALEINOPHOBIA
Die-das-ka-lee-no-foe-bee-ah
Often related to leaving the safety of one's parents and home, as well as going to school, this phobia cannot be directly traced to any Greek or Latin words.

CROSSING STREETS

AGYROPHOBIA
A-jy-ro-foe-bee-ah
or
DROMOPHOBIA
Drom-oh-foe-bee-ah
There is no Greek or Latin word that can explain the origin of agyrophobia. Dromophobia finds the origin of its meaning in *drome*, the Greek word for racecourse.

Related Phobias:
Motorphobia, fear of automobiles

CROWDS OR MOBS

DEMOPHOBIA
Dem-o-foe-bee-ah
or
OCHLOPHOBIA
Ok-lo-for-bee-ah
or
ENOCHLOPHOBIA,
Ee-nok-lo-foe-bee-ah
While there is no Greek or Latin word to trace the origin of enochlophobia, demophobia is derived from the Greek words *demo*, meaning people, and *mobil*, which means move. *Ochlo* is the Greek word for mob.

CROWDED PUBLIC PLACES

AGORAPHOBIA
Ag-or-a-foe-bee-ah
This common fear originates from the Greek word *agora*, meaning marketplace or open space. Extreme sufferers refuse to leave the safety of their own homes or familiar places.

HEARING GOOD NEWS

EUPHOBIA
You-foe-bee-ah
Taken from the Greek prefix *eu* meaning good or happy, this fear can also comprise an anxiety toward laughter and gaiety.

Related Phobias:
Cherophobia, fear of happiness

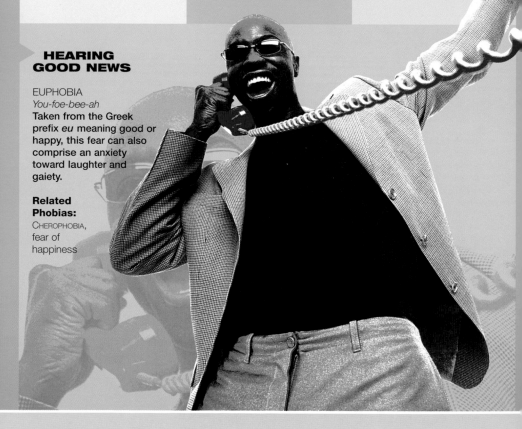

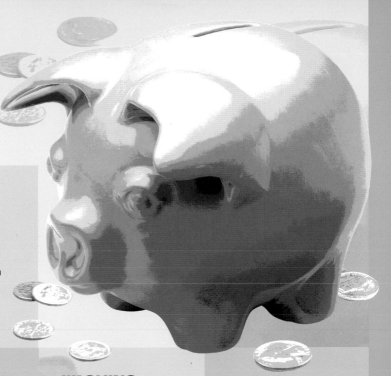

WEALTH

PLUTOPHOBIA
Plew-toe-foe-bee-ah
This term emanates from the Greek god of wealth and the underworld, *Pluto*.

POVERTY

PENIAPHOBIA
Pee-nee-ah-foe-bee-ah
***Penia* is the Greek word for insufficient or poor, which gives us the origin of this term.**

WASHING

ABLUTOPHOBIA
Ab-lew-toe-foe-bee-ah
Originating from the Latin verb to wash – *abluto* – this dread of washing extends to personal hygiene and also the fear of seeing others wash.

Related Phobias:
HYDROPHOBIA, fear of water

FINANCE

CHRIMATOPHOBIA
crim-at-oh-foe-bee-ah
This hatred of financial matters, whether personal or business, derives from the Greek word *chrima* meaning finance.

Related Phobias:
PENIAPHOBIA, fear of poverty

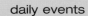

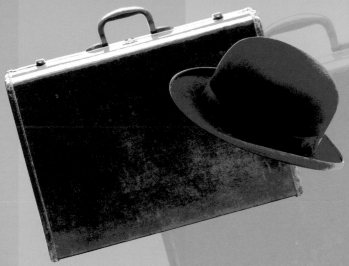

WORK

ERGOPHOBIA
Ur-go-foe-bee-ah
or
PONOPHOBIA
Pon-oh-foe-bee-ah
Derived from the Greek words *phobo* or *ergo*, both meaning work or toil, ergophobia relates to anxieties of failing to complete a task properly, whereas ponophobia is the fear or hatred of being tired through work.

Related Phobias:
Kopophobia, fear of fatigue

DUTY OR RESPONSIBILITY

PARALIPOPHOBIA
Pa-ra-li-po-foe-bee-ah
Derived from the Greek word *para*, meaning to protect, this phobia can relate to a fear of having or neglecting one's responsibilities.

Related Phobias:
Atelophobia, fear of imperfection

DECISIONS

DECIDOPHOBIA
Di-sy-do-foe-bee-ah
Taken loosely from the Latin word *judic*, meaning to judge, we may be able to explain the root of this word. Phobics of this disorder often suffer from low self-esteem, giving rise to indecision.

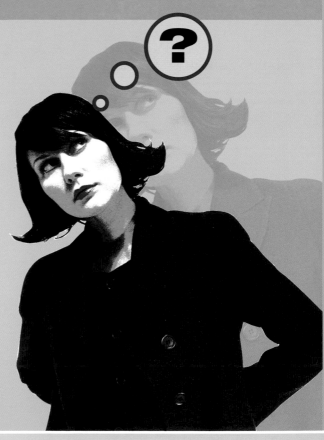

MOTION OR MOVEMENT

KINESOPHOBIA
Kin-ess-oh-foe-bee-ah
or
KINETOPHOBIA
Kin-et-oh-foe-bee-ah
Kine, the Greek word for movement, explains the origins of this commonly held fear by people who suffer motion sickness.

ANYTHING NEW

NEOPHOBIA
Nee-oh-foe-bee-ah
This fear of innovations and new surroundings is taken from the Greek word *neo*, meaning new or fresh.

Related Phobias:
TECHNOPHOBIA, fear of technology

MAKING CHANGES OR MOVING

TROPOPHOBIA
Trop-oh-foe-bee-ah
or
METATHESIOPHOBIA
Me-ta-thess-eo-foe-bee-ah
Tropophobia, anxiety about altering one's course, is rooted in the Greek *tropo*, meaning turn or bend. Metathesiophobia originates from the Greek *meta* – altered or changed.

DANCING

CHOROPHOBIA
Kor-oh-foe-bee-ah
Directly formed from the Greek verb *choro*, to dance, this phobia may also comprise an anxiety of being touched by someone of the opposite sex.

Related Phobias:
COITOPHOBIA, fear of sexual intercourse

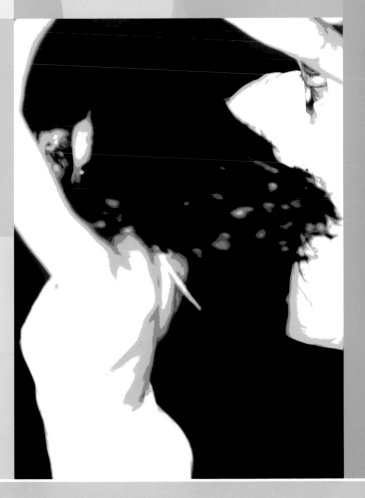

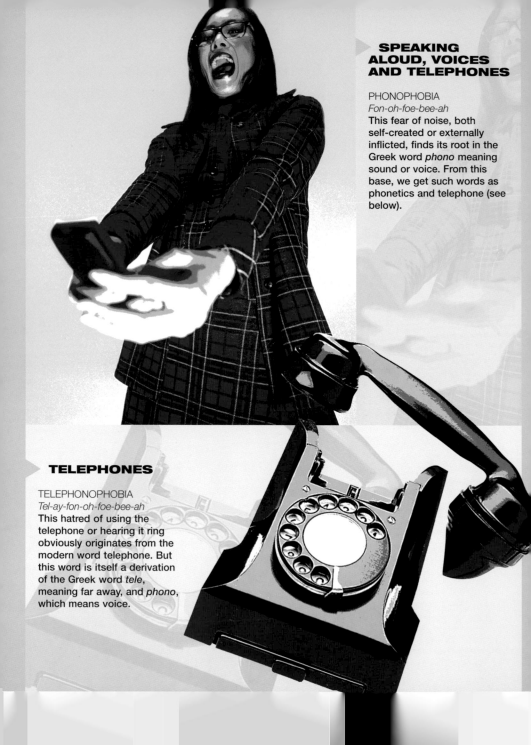

SPEAKING ALOUD, VOICES AND TELEPHONES

PHONOPHOBIA
Fon-oh-foe-bee-ah
This fear of noise, both self-created or externally inflicted, finds its root in the Greek word *phono* meaning sound or voice. From this base, we get such words as phonetics and telephone (see below).

TELEPHONES

TELEPHONOPHOBIA
Tel-ay-fon-oh-foe-bee-ah
This hatred of using the telephone or hearing it ring obviously originates from the modern word telephone. But this word is itself a derivation of the Greek word *tele*, meaning far away, and *phono*, which means voice.

RETURNING HOME

NOSTOPHOBIA
Nos-toe-foe-bee-ah
This dread of returning to one's dwelling place derives from the Greek word for abode – *nosto*.

PAPER

PAPYROPHOBIA
Pap-eye-row-foe-bee-ah
This dread can easily be traced to the Greek word *papyri*, meaning paper.

Related Phobias:
HEMOPHOBIA, fear of blood

HOME

ECOPHOBIA
Ee-ko-foe-bee-ah
Derived from the Greek word *eco*, meaning house, this fear encompasses not only household appliances but also anything else within the house.

HOME SURROUNDINGS

EICOPHOBIA
Eye-ko-foe-bee-ah

There is no direct Latin or Greek origin to this word's meaning. It most probably derives from the Greek word for house – *eco*.

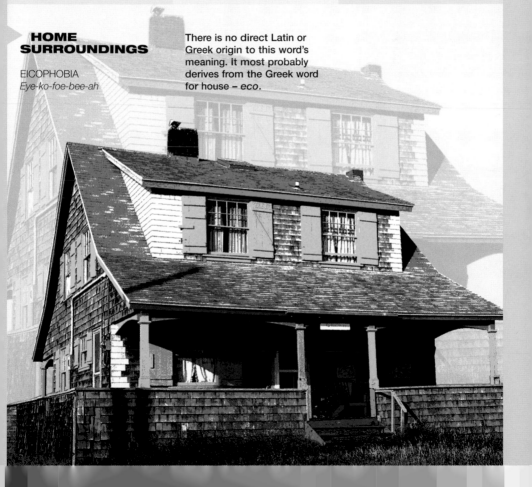

METAL

METALLOPHOBIA
Met-al-oh-foe-bee-ah
This word comes from the Greek word *metallo*, which means metal.

KNIVES

APOKOPHOBIA
a-pock-oh-foe-bee-ah
Apopkopto, the Greek word for cutting, gives us the origin of this dread of these kitchen carving implements.

GLASS

HYELOPHOBIA
Hi-yel-oh-foe-bee-ah
Hyalo is the Greek word for transparent or glass, which explains the origins of this word.

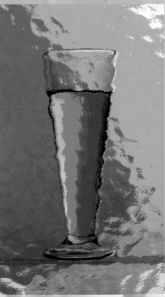

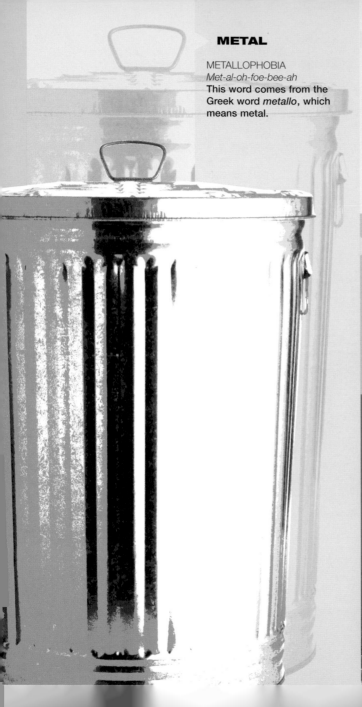

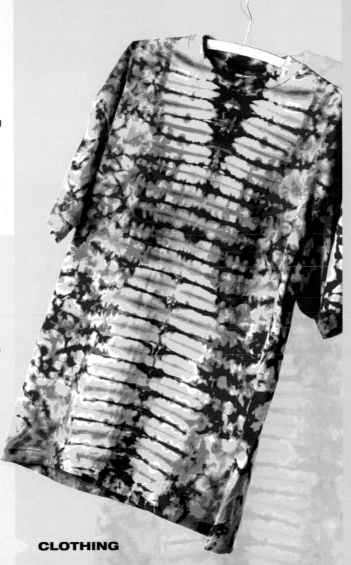

BEING ALONE

MONOPHOBIA
MON-OH-FOE-BEE-AH
or
AUTOPHOBIA
ort-oh-foe-bee-ah
While autophobia stems from
the Greek word *auto*, meaning
self, and relates to
a fear of one's own company,
monophobia can mean a fear
desolate places or a dread of
one's own company. Mono is
the Greek word for self.

GLARING LIGHTS

PHOTOAUGLIAPHOBIA
Fo-to-org-lee-a-foe-bee-ah
Photo is the Greek word for
light, which illuminates the
origins of this fear. Phobics of
this disorder dread the
thought of lights shining
directly upon their eyes.

Related Phobias:
NYCTOPHOBIA, fear of darkness

FLASHING LIGHTS

SELAPHOBIA
Cel-a-foe-bee-ah
There is no Greek or Latin
word that can help us trace
the origins of this term.

Related Phobias:
AURORAPHOBIA, fear of the
Northern Lights

CLOTHING

VESTIPHOBIA
Ve-sti-foe-bee-ah
Emanating from the Greek
word *vest*, meaning clothes,
this is the fear of one's own or
other peoples garments, as
well as certain fabrics.

Related Phobias:
GYMNOPHOBIA, fear of nudity

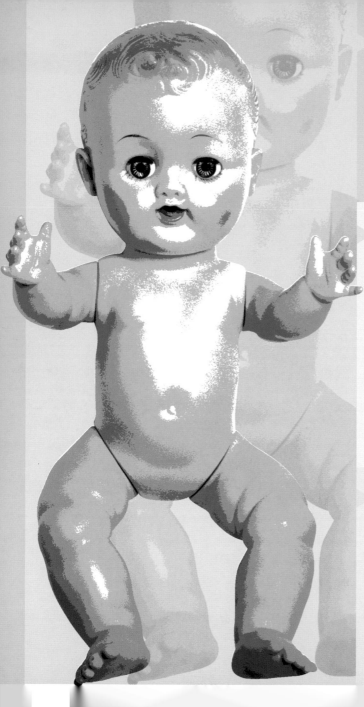

DOLLS

PEDIOPHOBIA
Ped-ee-oh-foe-bee-ah
Derived from the Greek word for child – *pedo* – this abnormal fear of dolls can also extend to a dread of infants. Not good news for parents.

PINS AND NEEDLES

AICHMOPHOBIA
Ay-ch-mo-foe-bee-ah
or
BELONEPHOBIA
Bel-on-ee-foe-bee-ah
The origin of aichmophobia derives in meaning from the Greek word *aichme*, meaning spear, and can also extend to a general dread of sharp things. *Belono* is the Greek word for needle, thus this phobia relates more specifically to needles.

PINS

ENETOPHOBIA
En-et-oh-foe-bee-ah
This fear of pins derives from the Greek word *eneto*, meaning injection.

CLOCKS

CHRONOMENTROPHOBIA
Kro-no-men-tro-foe-bee-ah
This fear of clocks derives from the Greek god *Chronos*, who was sometimes referred to as Father Time, from which comes the Greek word *chrono*, meaning time.

CLOCKS OR TIME

CHRONOPHOBIA
Kro-no-foe-bee-ah
Originating from the Greek word *chrono*, meaning time, this dread is often experienced by prison inmates and characterized by claustrophobia.

Related Phobias:
GERASCOPHOBIA, fear of growing old

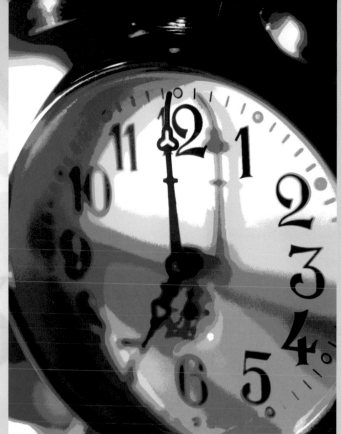

CRYSTALS OR GLASS

CRYSTALLOPHOBIA
Crys-tal-oh-foe-bee-ah
This dread of crystals originates from the Greek word *crystallo*, which means glass or crystal.

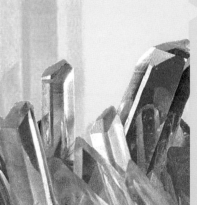

PROPERTY

DOMATOPHOBIA
Dom-at-oh-foe-bee-ah
This fear of being in one's own home or of being confined is directly derived from the Greek word for house – *domo*.

Related Phobias:
AUROPHOBIA, fear of materialism

VENTRILOQUISTS DUMMIES OR WAX STATUES

AUTOMATONOPHOBIA
or-tom-a-ton-oh-foe-bee-ah
Although there is no direct Greek or Latin word to explain the word automaton, it is interesting to note that the Greek word *auto* means directed from the inside.

PUPPETS

PUPAPHOBIA
Pew-pa-foe-bee-ah
This dread of dolls and puppets derives from the Greek word *pupa*, meaning small girl or puppet.

MIRRORS OR SEEING ONESELF IN A MIRROR

EISOPTROPHOBIA
Ee-sop-tro-foe-bee-ah
This phobia originates from the Greek word *eisoptro*, meaning mirror.

Related Phobias:
DYSMORPHOBIA, fear of looking in the mirror because one's reflection presents a figure of ugliness

MIRRORS

CATOPTROPHOBIA
Cat-op-tro-foe-bee-ah
This fear derives in meaning from the Greek word *catoptro* meaning mirror.

SMALL OBJECTS

TAPINOPHOBIA
Tap-in-oh-foe-bee-ah
Tapino is the Greek word for low, which explains the origins of this phobia.

CERTAIN FABRICS

TEXTOPHOBIA
Tex-toe-foe-bee-ah
There is no Greek or Latin word that can directly explain the origins of this word. It is probably derived from the modern word, texture.

STRING

LINONOPHOBIA
Lin-on-oh-foe-bee-ah
The fear of string comes from the Greek word *lino*, which translates as cord or thread.

Related Phobias:
MERINTHOPHOBIA, fear of being tied up

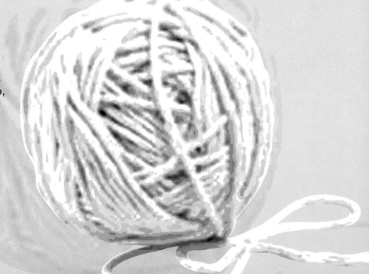

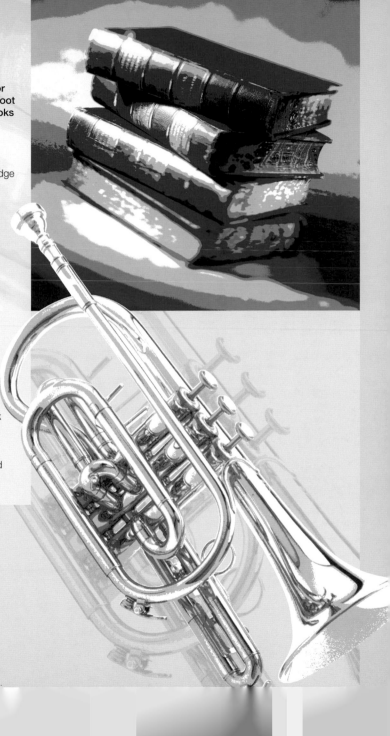

BOOKS

BIBLIOPHOBIA
Bib-li-oh-foe-bee-ah
Biblio is the Greek word for book, which explains the root meaning of this fear of books often through one's own illiteracy.

Related Phobias:
GNOSIOPHOBIA, fear of knowledge

FLUTES

AULOPHOBIA
or-lo-foe-bee-ah
This fear of flutes and wind instruments derives in meaning from the Greek word for wind – *aello*.

Related Phobias:
ANEMOPHOBIA, fear of the wind

MUSIC

MELOPHOBIA
Mel-oh-foe-bee-ah
This strong dislike of music derives from the Greek word *ode*, meaning song. From this we also get the commonly-used word, melody.

RAZORS

XYROPHOBIA
Zy-ro-foe-bee-ah
This anxiety can be directly
traced in origin to the Greek
word *xyro*, meaning razor.

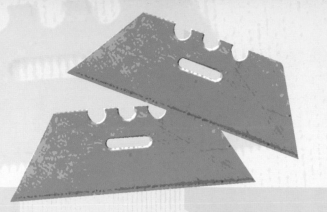

MONEY

CHROMETOPHOBIA
Kro-met-oh-foe-bee-ah
or
CHREMATOPHOBIA
Cre-mat-oh-foe-bee-ah
Chremato is the Greek
verb to transact or trade,
which explains the origins
of this vehement distaste
for money. Some sufferers
may fear catching germs
from well-handled coins.

BEDS OR
GOING TO BED

CLINOPHOBIA
Clin-oh-foe-bee-ah
Emanating from the Greek
word for bed – *clino* – this
excessive anxiety can
comprise a dread of beds,
nightmares, bedwetting,
insomnia, and even the fear
of never waking up again.

Related Phobias:
ONEIROPHOBIA, fear of dreams

DINING
OR DINNER
CONVERSATIONS

DEIPNOPHOBIA
De-ip-no-foe-bee-ah
This unusual fear of talking
while eating, or meal
conversations in general,
finds its origin in the Greek
word *deipno*, which means
dinner.

Related Phobias:
GLOSSOPHOBIA, fear of speaking
in public

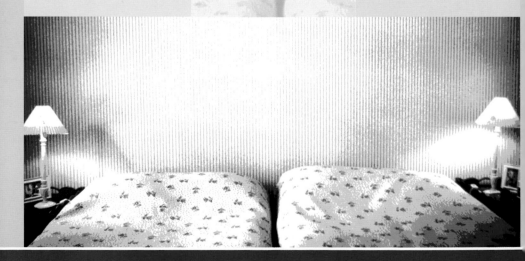

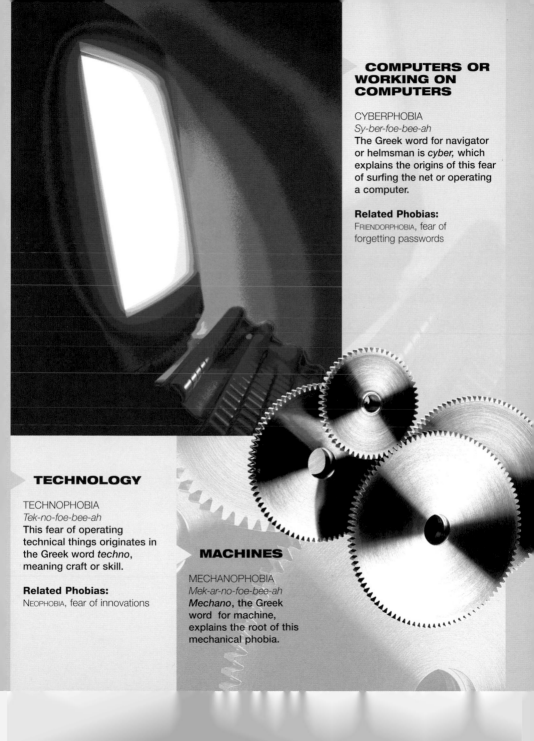

COMPUTERS OR WORKING ON COMPUTERS

CYBERPHOBIA
Sy-ber-foe-bee-ah
The Greek word for navigator or helmsman is *cyber,* which explains the origins of this fear of surfing the net or operating a computer.

Related Phobias:
FRIENDORPHOBIA, fear of forgetting passwords

TECHNOLOGY

TECHNOPHOBIA
Tek-no-foe-bee-ah
This fear of operating technical things originates in the Greek word *techno,* meaning craft or skill.

Related Phobias:
NEOPHOBIA, fear of innovations

MACHINES

MECHANOPHOBIA
Mek-ar-no-foe-bee-ah
Mechano, the Greek word for machine, explains the root of this mechanical phobia.

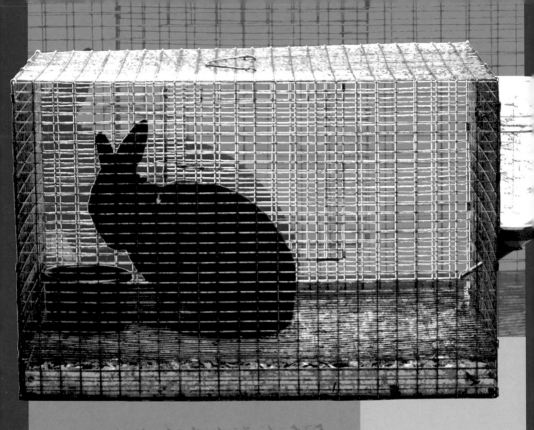

LOCKED IN AN ENCLOSED PLACE

CLEISIOPHOBIA
Cly-sio-foe-bee-ah
or
CLEITHROPHOBIA
Cly-thro-foe-bee-ah
or
CLITHROPHOBIA
Cli-thro-foe-bee-ah

All three phobias derive from *cleithro*, the Greek verb to shut, and pertain to a fear of being locked in as opposed to being in a confined space.

CONFINED SPACES

CLAUSTROPHOBIA
Kloss-tro-foe-bee-ah
This is the most common phobia, experienced worldwide, which emanates from the Latin word *claustro*, meaning shut or lock.

Related Phobias:
DOMATOPHOBIA, fear of being locked in a house

VERTIGO WHEN LOOKING DOWN

ILLYNGOPHOBIA
Ill-in-go-foe-bee-ah
There are no Greek or Latin words to explain the origins of this term.

OPEN HIGH PLACES

AEROACROPHOBIA
Air-oh-ac-row-foe-bee-ah
The Greek words *aero*, meaning air, and *acro*, which means highest, form the root meaning of this fear of elevation.

OPEN SPACES

AGORAPHOBIA
Ag-or-ah-foe-bee-ah
Commonly accepted to be the most widespread phobia, this fear of open spaces and crowds derives in meaning from the Greek word for marketplace – *agora*.

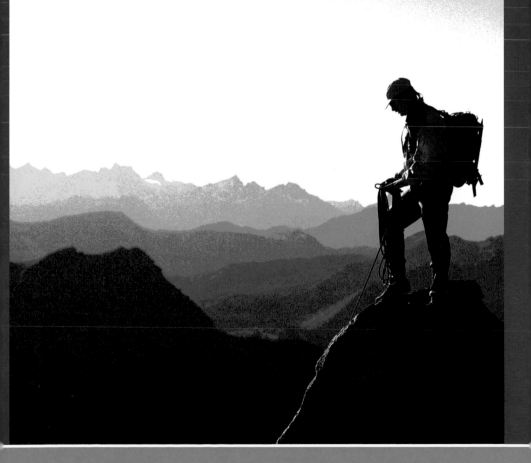

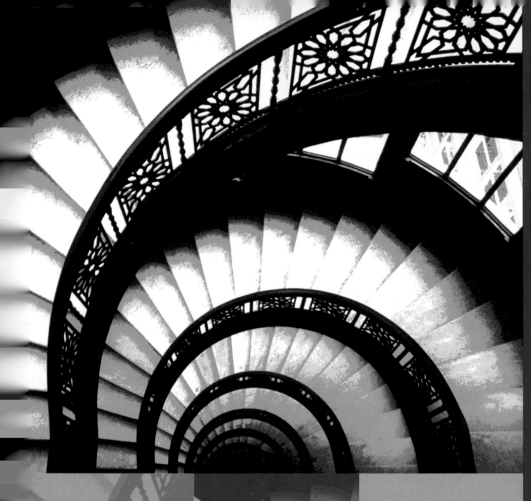

STAIRS OR CLIMBING STAIRS

CLIMACOPHOBIA
Cly-mac-oh-foe-bee-ah
There are no Greek or Latin words that can help us trace the origin of this word.

STAIRWAYS

BATHMOPHOBIA
Ba-thur-mo-foe-bee-ah
This unusual phobia originates from the Greek word for stairs or steps – *bathmo*.

DIZZINESS OR WHIRLPOOLS

DINOPHOBIA
Dye-no-foe-bee-ah
This unsettling anxiety derives in meaning from the Greek word *dino*, meaning whirling or full of eddies.

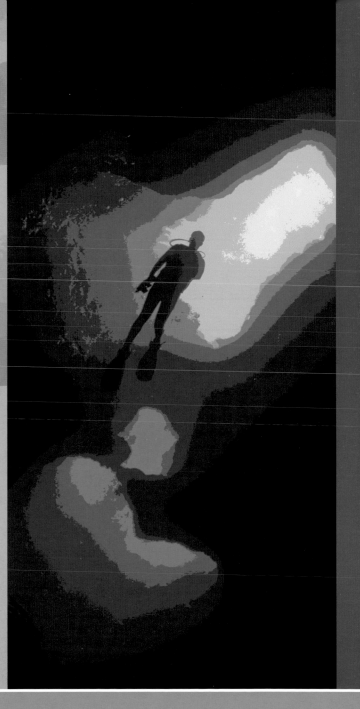

DEPTHS

BATHOPHOBIA
Ba-tho-foe-bee-ah
Often associated with wells or descending into them, this fear of depths takes its name from the Greek word *batho*, meaning depth.

Related Phobias:
ABLUTOPHOBIA, fear of bathing

BEING IN GLOOMY OR DARK PLACES

LYGOPHOBIA
Lie-go-foe-bee-ah
The Greek word *lygo* means shadow or darkness, which explains the origin of this term.

Related Phobias:
NYCTOPHOBIA, fear of darkness

LARGE THINGS

MEGALOPHOBIA
Meg-a-low-foe-bee-ah
This fear of large objects finds its origin in the Greek word *mega*, meaning enormous or powerful. This is also the root of such modern terms as megalomaniac and megalopolis.

NARROW THINGS OR PLACES

STENOPHOBIA
Sten-oh-foe-bee-ah
Steno is the Greek word for narrow, which explains the origins of this word.

Related Phobias:

CLAUSTROPHOBIA, fear of small spaces

NARROWNESS

ANGINOPHOBIA
An-ji-no-foe-bee-ah
This fear of narrowness, and therefore restriction, also relates to a dread of heartburn or angina, and takes its name from the Greek word *angio*, meaning blood vessel.

Related Phobias:

PNIGOPHOBIA, fear of choking

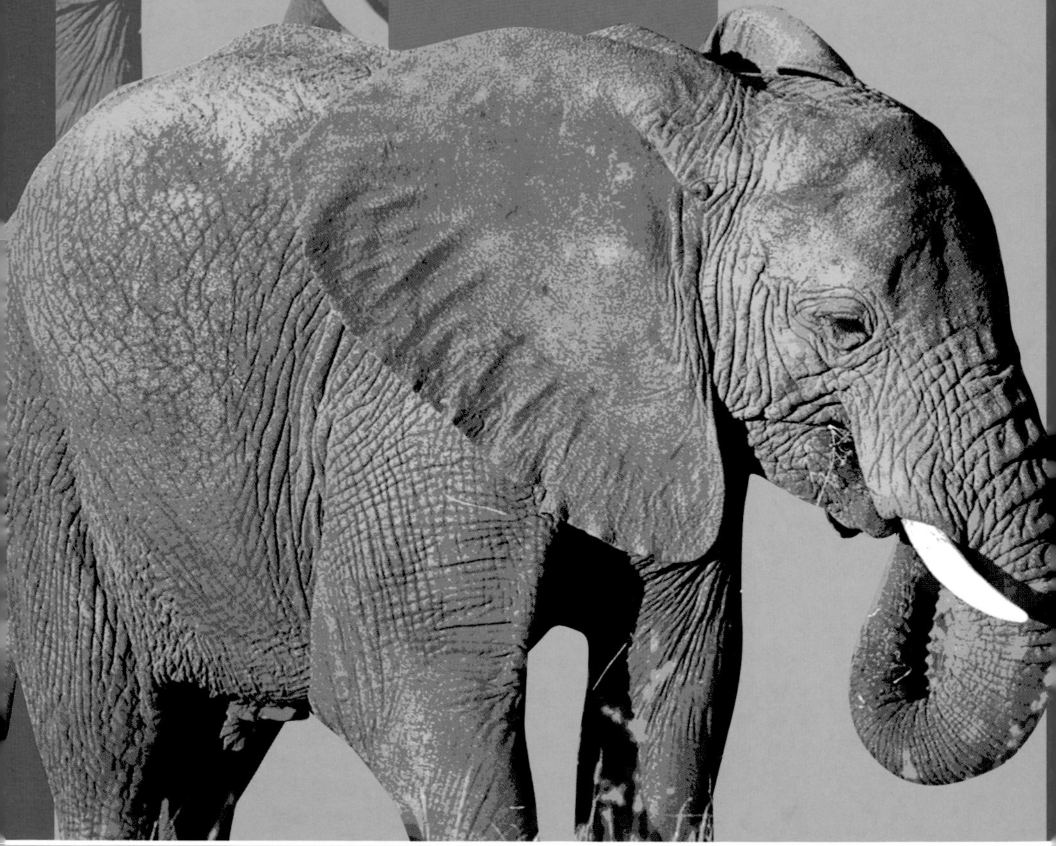

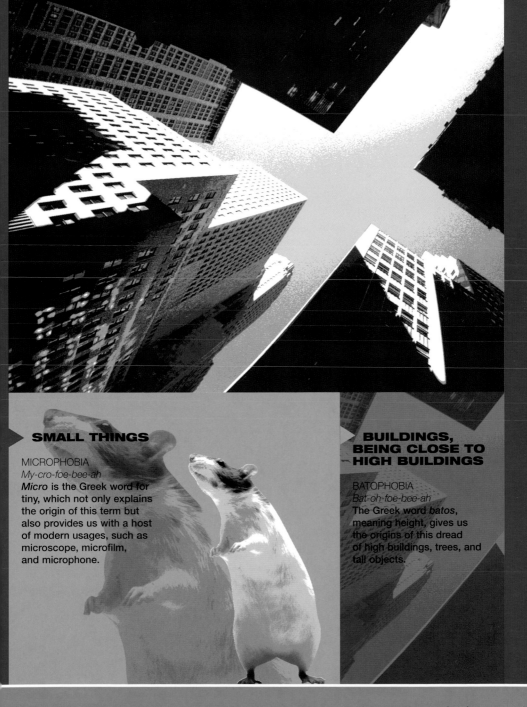

SMALL THINGS

MICROPHOBIA
My-cro-foe-bee-ah
Micro is the Greek word for tiny, which not only explains the origin of this term but also provides us with a host of modern usages, such as microscope, microfilm, and microphone.

BUILDINGS, BEING CLOSE TO HIGH BUILDINGS

BATOPHOBIA
Bat-oh-foe-bee-ah
The Greek word *batos*, meaning height, gives us the origins of this dread of high buildings, trees, and tall objects.

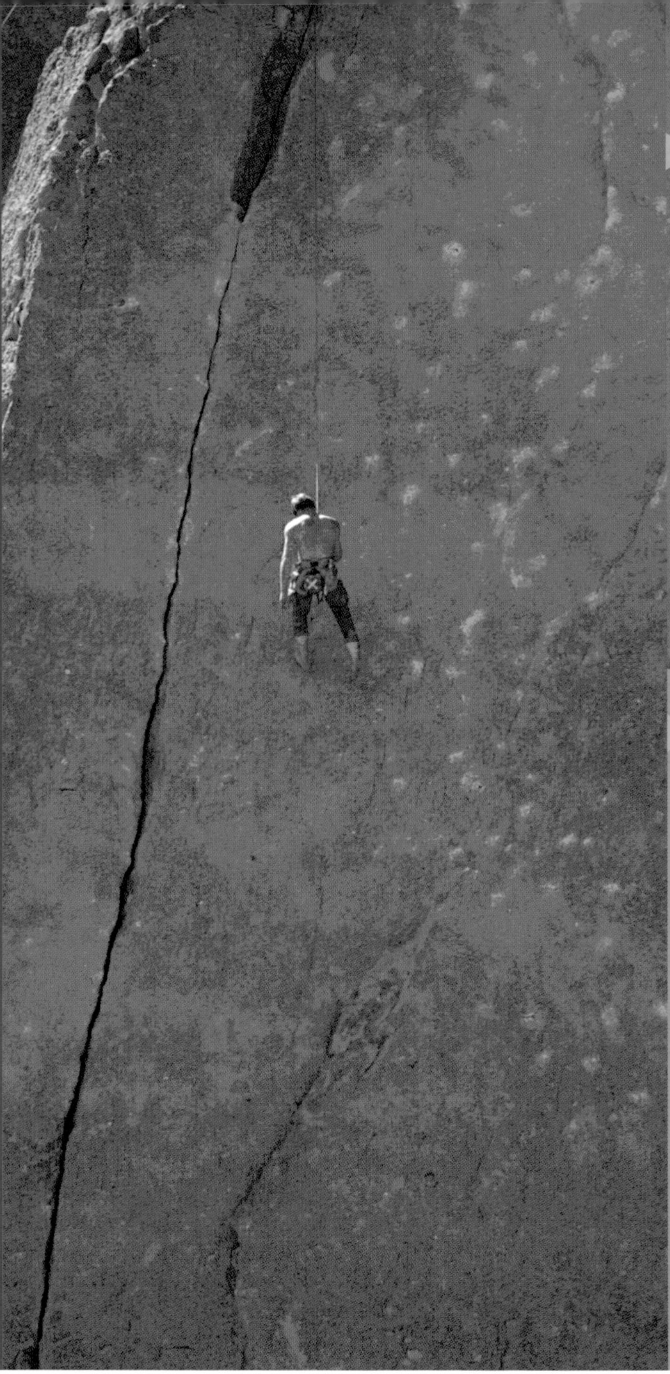

▶ PRECIPICES

CREMNOPHOBIA
Krem-no-foe-bee-ah
**The Greek word for precipice
or cliff is *cremno*, and
therefore explains the word
origin of this common fear.**

Related Phobias:
CATAPEDAPHOBIA, fear of jumping
from high places

▶ HEIGHTS

ACROPHOBIA
Ac-row-foe-bee-ah
or
ALTOPHOBIA
Al-toe-foe-bee-ah
or
HYPOSOPHOBIA
Hi-po-so-foe-bee-ah
***Acro* is the Greek word for
highest point or top, while
alto is the Latin equivalent.
Both refer to a terror of high
places. *Hypo* is the Greek
prefix for that which lies
beneath or under
and usually relates to
a fear of acrobatics.**

Related Phobias:
BATOPHOBIA, being close to
high buildings

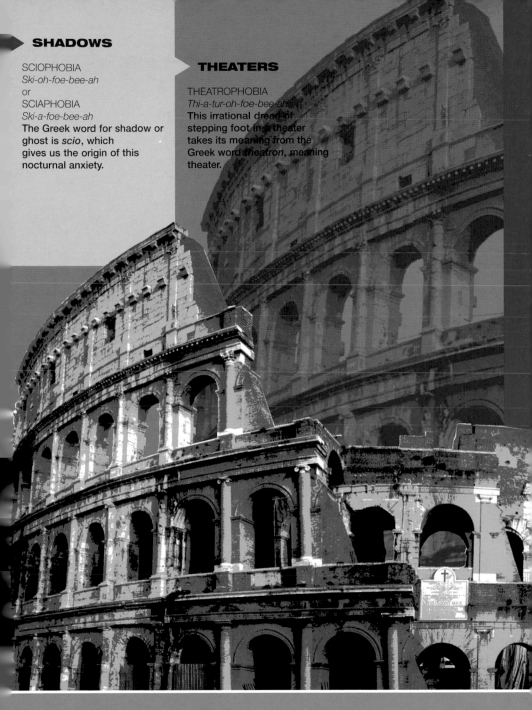

SHADOWS

SCIOPHOBIA
Ski-oh-foe-bee-ah
or
SCIAPHOBIA
Ski-a-foe-bee-ah
The Greek word for shadow or ghost is *scio*, which gives us the origin of this nocturnal anxiety.

THEATERS

THEATROPHOBIA
Thi-a-tur-oh-foe-bee-ah
This irrational dread of stepping foot in a theater takes its meaning from the Greek word *theatron*, meaning theater.

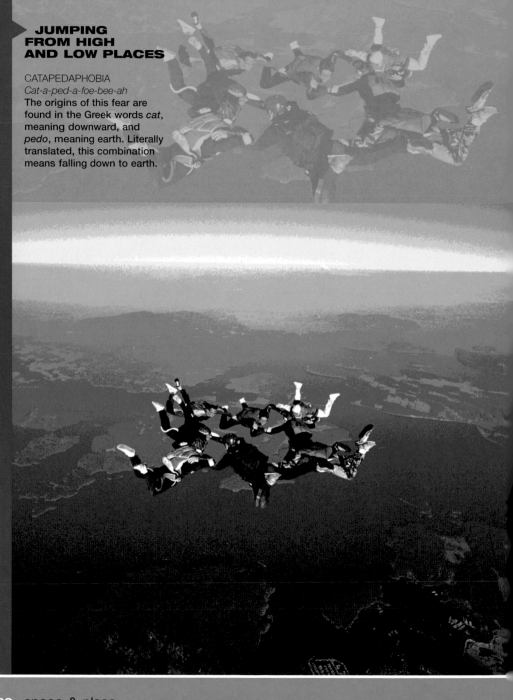

JUMPING FROM HIGH AND LOW PLACES

CATAPEDAPHOBIA
Cat-a-ped-a-foe-bee-ah
The origins of this fear are found in the Greek words *cat*, meaning downward, and *pedo*, meaning earth. Literally translated, this combination means falling down to earth.

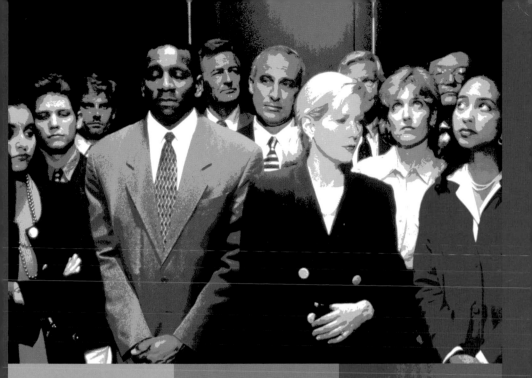

CERTAIN PLACES

TOPOPHOBIA
Top-oh-foe-bee-ah
This fear of certain places, often used to describe stage fright originates from the Greek word *topo*, meaning place or region.

Related Phobias:
THEATROPHOBIA, fear of theaters

EMPTY ROOMS

CENOPHOBIA
Sen-oh-foe-bee-ah
or
CENTOPHOBIA
Sen-to-foe-bee-ah
This dread of empty rooms or places takes its meaning from the Greek word *ceno*, which translates as empty.

Related Phobias:
MONOPHOBIA, fear of being left alone

CROWDED ROOMS

KOINONIPHOBIA
Coy-non-ee-foe-bee-ah
Derived from the Greek word *coino*, meaning shared or common, this phobia exhibits itself in a room full of people.

Related Phobias:
SOCIOPHOBIA, fear of people

RIDING IN A CAR OR VEHICLE

AMAXOPHOBIA
Am-ax-o-foe-bee-ah
This restrictive fear of traveling finds its word origin in the Greek word for vehicle or wagon – *amaxo*.

AUTOMOBILES

MOTORPHOBIA
Mo-tor-foe-bee-ah
The Greek word *moto* means to move, and therefore provides us with not only the origin of this term, but also key words such as motorcar and motivate.

BEING IN A MOVING AUTOMOBILE

OCHOPHOBIA
O-cho-foe-bee-ah
It is safe to presume that there were not many cars in ancient Greece or Rome, therefore we cannot trace the origin of this fear to these times.

ROAD TRAVEL OR TRAVEL

HODOPHOBIA
Hod-o-foe-bee-ah

Hodo is the Greek word for way or path, which succinctly explains the origins of this term.

AIRSICKNESS

AERONAUSIPHOBIA
Air-o-nor-si-foe-bee-ah
The Greek words *aero*, meaning air, and *naus*, which means sailor, literally translate as sea and air, to describe this dreaded fear of being sick on airplanes. Such a condition is often experienced by people who have no sea legs.

Related Phobias:
AEROPHOBIA, fear of the air or wind

BICYCLES

CYCLOPHOBIA
Si-klo-foe-bee-ah
This peculiar fear of bicycles emanates from the Greek word *cyclo* meaning round or circular.

SPEED

TACHOPHOBIA
Tak-o-foe-bee-ah
The origin of this term can be found in the Greek word *tacho*, meaning swift or rapid.

Related Phobias:
KINESOPHOBIA, fear of motion

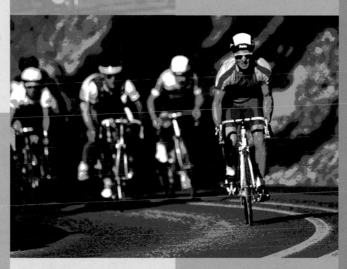

STREETS

AGYROPHOBIA
A-jy-ro-foe-bee-ah
The Greek word *gyro*, meaning spinning or whirling, may hold some clues to the origin of this fear of traffic and streets in general.

CROSSING STREETS

DROMOPHOBIA
Drom-oh-foe-bee-ah
This unfortunate phobia finds the origin of its meaning in *drome*, the Greek word for racecourse.

Related Phobias:
MOTORPHOBIA, fear of automobiles

BRIDGES OR CROSSING THEM

GEPHYROPHOBIA
Jef-ee-row-foe-bee-ah
Gephyro is the Greek word for bridge, which gives us a clear explanation of how this fear was named. Sufferers of this phobia are unable to go near a bridge, by foot or in a car.

FLYING

AVIOPHOBIA
A-vi-o-foe-bee-ah
or
AVIATOPHOBIA
A-vi-ay-toe-foe-bee-ah
or
PTEROMERHANOPHOBIA
Ter-o-mu-ran-o-foe-bee-ah
Avi is the Latin word for bird, while *ptero* is Greek for feather or wing.

Related Phobias:
EMETOPHOBIA, fear of vomiting

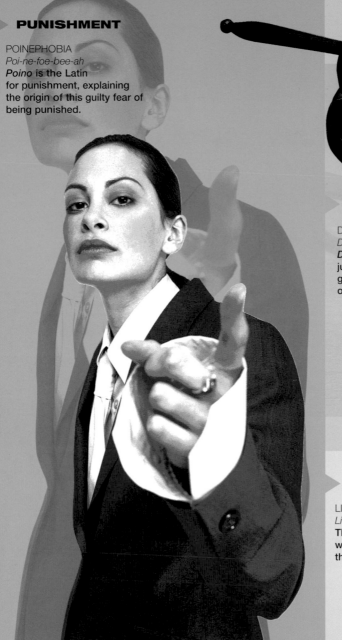

PUNISHMENT

POINEPHOBIA
Poi-ne-foe-bee-ah
Poino is the Latin for punishment, explaining the origin of this guilty fear of being punished.

JUSTICE

DIKEPHOBIA
Dy-ke-foe-bee-ah
Diko is the Greek word for justice or manner, which gives us the root of this fear of justice.

LAWSUITS

LITICAPHOBIA
Lit-ik-a-foe-bee-ah
There are no Greek or Latin words to explain the origins of this very commonplace fear.

RAPE

VIRGINITIPHOBIA
Vir-jin-it-oh-foe-bee-ah
This anxiety derives in
meaning from the Latin word
virgo meaning maiden, fragile
twig, or shoot.

Related Phobias:
AUTOMYSOPHOBIA, fear of
being dirty

STEALING

CLEPTOPHOBIA
Clep-toe-foe-bee-ah
or
KLEPTOPHOBIA
Klep-toe-foe-bee-ah
This fear of having one's
property stolen or of
becoming a thief, finds its
origin in the Greek word

klepto, meaning thief, theft, or
steal. From this we also
obtain the modern usage,
kleptomaniac.

Related Phobias:
XENONOSOCOMIOPHOBIA, fear
of foreign pickpockets

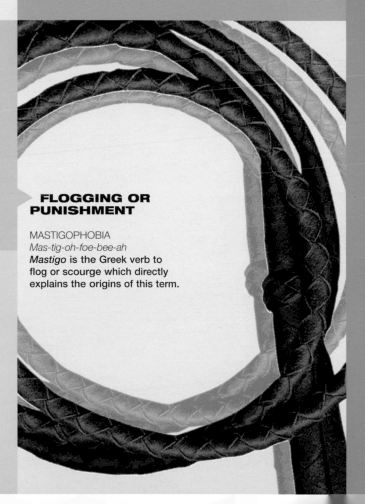

BEING BOUND
OR TIED UP

MERINTHOPHOBIA
Mur-in-tho-foe-bee-ah
The Greek word for string is
merintho, which provides us
with an easy explanation of
where this word comes from.

Related Phobias:
LINONOPHOBIA, hatred of string

FLOGGING OR
PUNISHMENT

MASTIGOPHOBIA
Mas-tig-oh-foe-bee-ah
Mastigo is the Greek verb to
flog or scourge which directly
explains the origins of this term.

BEING HARMED
BY WICKED MEN
OR BURGLARS

SCELEROPHOBIA
Skel-er-oh-foe-bee-ah
This dread derives from the
Latin word *scelero*, meaning
evil deed.

Related Phobias:
THANATOPHOBIA, fear of death

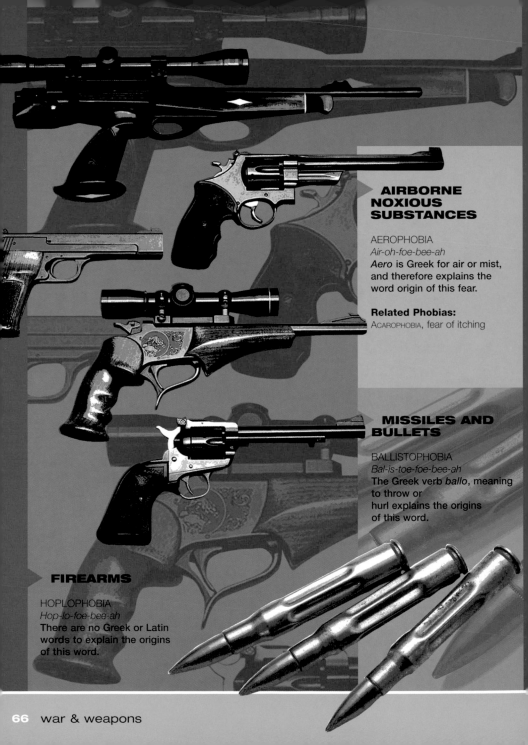

AIRBORNE NOXIOUS SUBSTANCES

AEROPHOBIA
Air-oh-foe-bee-ah
Aero is Greek for air or mist, and therefore explains the word origin of this fear.

Related Phobias:
ACAROPHOBIA, fear of itching

MISSILES AND BULLETS

BALLISTOPHOBIA
Bal-is-toe-foe-bee-ah
The Greek verb *ballo*, meaning to throw or hurl explains the origins of this word.

FIREARMS

HOPLOPHOBIA
Hop-lo-foe-bee-ah
There are no Greek or Latin words to explain the origins of this word.

RADIATION

RADIOPHOBIA
Ray-deo-foe-bee-ah
This anxiety of radiation can also extend to x-ray machines and takes its meaning from the Greek word *radio*, meaning to radiate.

NUCLEAR WEAPONS

NUCLEOMITUPHOBIA
Nu-cle-om-it-yew-foe-bee-ah
There is no Latin or Greek word which can trace the origins of this modern term, since nuclear science is clearly a modern phenomenon.

Related Phobias:
CERAUNOPHOBIA, fear of thunder

ATOMIC EXPLOSIONS

ATOMOSOPHOBIA
At-om-os-oh-foe-bee-ah
Obviously the Greeks and Romans were not privy to atomic science so there is no ancient word to trace the origins of this term.

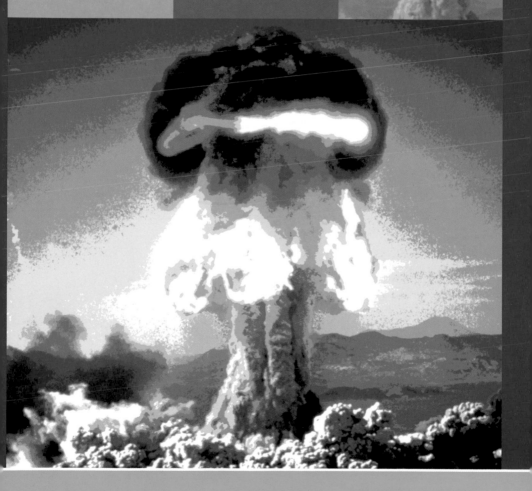

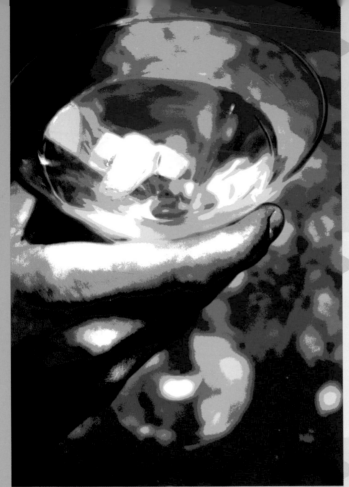

DRINKING

DIPSOPHOBIA
Dip-so-foe-bee-ah
This intense fear of drinking derives from the Greek word *dipso*, meaning thirsty.

Related Phobias:
DIPLOPHOBIA, fear of double vision

EATING OR SWALLOWING

PHAGOPHOBIA
Fag-oh-foe-bee-ah
This fear of eating finds its meaning in the Greek verb *phago*, meaning to consume.

Related Phobias:
ANGINOPHOBIA, fear of choking

WINE

OENOPHOBIA
Ee-no-foe-bee-ah
This irrational dread of wine finds the root of its meaning in the Greek translation of the word – *oeino*.

Related Phobias:
METHYPHOBIA, fear of becoming alcoholic.

ALCOHOL

METHYPHOBIA
Me-thi-foe-bee-ah
or
POTOPHOBIA
Pot-o-foe-bee-ah
Stemming from the Greek word *methyl*, meaning alcohol, methyphobia relates to a fear of becoming dependent on alcohol. Similarly *poto* is the Latin word for drink and relates to a general fear of drinking.

Related Phobias:
TURISTAPHOBIA, fear of having a bad stomach from something one has drunk

MEAT

CARNOPHOBIA
Car-no-foe-bee-ah
Carne is the Latin word for meat or flesh. This anxiety extends to both cooked and raw meat.

GARLIC

ALLIUMPHOBIA
Al-lee-um-foe-bee-ah
This fear of garlic can also extend to other pungent vegetables. *Allium* is the Latin word for garlic.

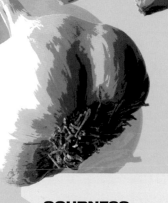

EATING OR DRINKING

SITOPHOBIA
Sy-toe-foe-bee-ah
An intense fear of eating and drinking, sitophobia finds its origins in the Greek word *sito*, meaning food.

FOOD

CIBOPHOBIA
Si-bo-foe-bee-ah
Cibo is Latin word for food. This irrational dread is directed toward specific types of food, the consuming of which can result in vomiting and nausea.

Related Phobias:
GEUMAPHOBIA, fear of taste

SOURNESS

ACEROPHOBIA
A-ser-oh-foe-bee-ah
This fear of bitter things finds its root in the Latin word for sour, *acerbo*. From this we also derive the modern term acerbic, meaning sharp or bitter.

PEANUT BUTTER STICKING TO THE ROOF OF ONE'S MOUTH

ARACHIBUTYROPHOBIA
A-rak-ee-but-yur-oh-foe-bee-ah
Originating from the Greek word for peanut – *araki*, this phobia can also relate to a fear of swallowing or choking.

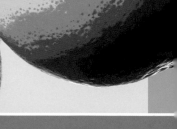

COOKING

MAGEIROCOPHOBIA
Ma-jir-oh-coe-foe-bee-ah
There is no Latin or Greek word to directly explain the origin of this fear of cooking for others.

POLITICIANS

POLITICOPHOBIA
Pol-it-e-ko-foe-bee-ah
This hatred of politicians
originates from the Greek
word *polis*, meaning city or
body of government.

RELATIVES

SYNGENESOPHOBIA
Sin-gen-ess-oh-foe-bee-ah
This hatred of one's relatives
derives from the Latin word
syn, meaning united, and the
Greek word *genus*, meaning
race or class.

STEPMOTHER

NOVERCAPHOBIA
No-ver-ka-foe-bee-ah
Novercalis, the Latin word for
stepmother explains the
origin of this word.

BUMS OR BEGGARS

HOBOPHOBIA
Hoe-bow-foe-bee-ah
There is no Greek or Latin
word to explain the origin of
this phobia of tramps and
beggars, however the term
probably derives from the
American vernacular *hobo*,
meaning vagrant.

MOTHER-IN-LAW

PENTHERAPHOBIA
Pen-th-ra-foe-bee-ah
This hatred of being around
one's mother-in-law is directly
derived from the Greek word
for the same, *penthera*.

Related Phobias:
WICCAPHOBIA, fear of witches

STEPFATHER

VITRICOPHOBIA
Vit-ri-co-foe-bee-ah
This common dislike
originates in meaning
from the Latin word for
stepfather – *vetrico*.

GOING BALD

PHALACROPHOBIA
Fal-ak-ro-foe-bee-ah
This fear of losing one's hair
derives directly from the
Greek word *phalacro*,
meaning smooth.

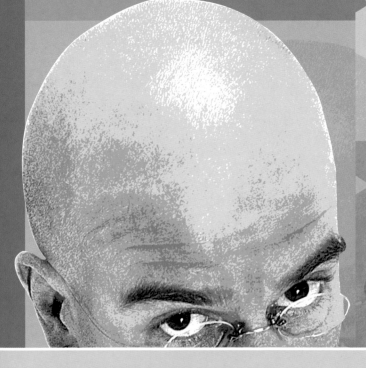

BALD PEOPLE

PELADOPHOBIA
Pe-lad-oh-foe-bee-ah
There is no Greek or Latin
word to explain the derivation
of this fear of bald people, or
becoming bald.

Related Phobias:
CHAETOPHOBIA, hatred of hair

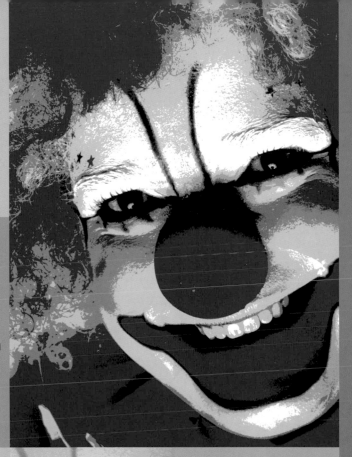

PARENTS-IN-LAW

SOCERAPHOBIA
Sok-er-a-foe-bee-ah
This common dread of one's in-laws originates from the Latin word for father-in-law – *soceri*.

Related Phobias:
PARALIPOPHOBIA, fear of responsibility

BEARING A DEFORMED CHILD OR DEFORMED PEOPLE

TERATOPHOBIA
Ter-at-o-foe-bee-ah
This common anxiety directly originates from the Greek word *terato*, which means monster or malformation.

Related Phobias:
CALIYGNEPHOBIA, fear of beautiful women

PROSTITUTES OR VENEREAL DISEASE

CYPRIDOPHOBIA
Sip-rid-oh-foe-bee-ah
An excessive fear of catching sexual diseases, or contact with a prostitute, this phobia finds its origin in the Greek word *cyprid*, meaning a lewd or licentious woman.

Related Phobias:
SCABIOPHOBIA, fear of catching scabies

CLOWNS

COULROPHOBIA
Ku-le-row-foe-bee-ah

There is no Latin or Greek word to trace the origin of this dread of clowns.

ROBBERS OR BEING ROBBED

HARPAXOPHOBIA
Har-pax-oh-foe-bee-ah
There is no Greek or Latin word to explain the derivation of this term. However, Harpies, the mythical winged creatures who used to filch food from sailors, may hold some clues.

Related Phobias:
SCELEROPHOBIA, fear of wicked people

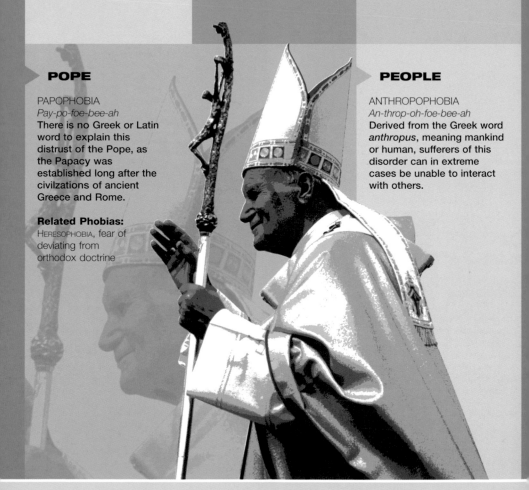

THE OPPOSITE SEX

HETEROPHOBIA
Het-er-oh-foe-bee-ah
or
SEXOPHPOBIA
Sex-oh-foe-bee-ah
Hetero is the Greek word for other, while *sex* is the Latin word for division. This explains these fears of the opposite sex and the modern usage of heterosexual.

TEENAGERS

EPHEBIPHOBIA
Eff-eb-ee-foe-bee-ah
This fear of teenagers originates in meaning from the Greek word *hebe*, meaning pubescent or youthful.

Related Phobias:
PHONOPHOBIA, fear of noise

YOUNG GIRLS OR VIRGINS

PARTHENOPHOBIA
Par-then-oh-foe-bee-ah
Partho, the Greek word for virgin, explains the origins of this term. Sufferers of this phobia cannot stand to be in the company of young girls.

Related Phobias:
PARAPHOBIA, fear of sexual perversion

POPE

PAPOPHOBIA
Pay-po-foe-bee-ah
There is no Greek or Latin word to explain this distrust of the Pope, as the Papacy was established long after the civilzations of ancient Greece and Rome.

Related Phobias:
HERESOPHOBIA, fear of deviating from orthodox doctrine

PEOPLE

ANTHROPOPHOBIA
An-throp-oh-foe-bee-ah
Derived from the Greek word *anthropus*, meaning mankind or human, sufferers of this disorder can in extreme cases be unable to interact with others.

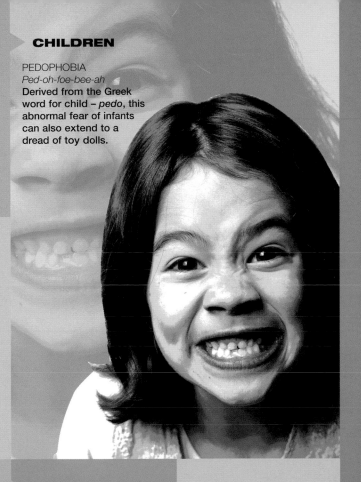

BEARDS

POGONOPHOBIA
Pog-on-oh-foe-bee-ah
This dread of beards or facial hair evolves from the Greek word *pogo*, for beard.

Related Phobias:
GENIOPHOBIA, fear of chins

MEN

ANDROPHOBIA
An-dro-foe-bee-ah
or
HOMINOPHOBIA
Hom-in-oh-foe-bee-ah
Hominophobia derives from the Latin word for man – *homo. Androis*, the Greek word for masculine, explains the origins of this term describing a fear of men.

CHILDREN

PEDOPHOBIA
Ped-oh-foe-bee-ah
Derived from the Greek word for child – *pedo*, this abnormal fear of infants can also extend to a dread of toy dolls.

WOMEN

GYNOPHOBIA
Guy-no-foe-bee-ah
or
GYNEPHOBIA
Guy-ne-foe-bee-ah
Gyno is the Greek word for woman, and so the origins of this excessive hatred of the fairer sex.

PEOPLE IN GENERAL OR SOCIETY

SOCIOPHOBIA
So-shi-oh-foe-bee-ah
Socio is the Latin word for companion, making the origins of this fear of friendship clear.

Related Phobias:
SYMBIOPHOBIA, fear of intimacy

TYRANTS

TYRANNOPHOBIA
Ty-ran-oh-foe-bee-ah
This hatred of dictators emanates from the Latin word *tyranni*, meaning oppressor.

Related Phobias:
RHABDOPHOBIA, fear of punishment

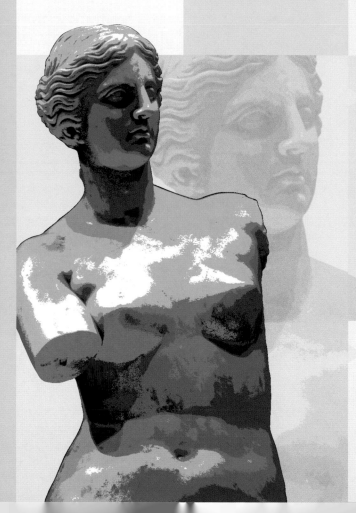

JEWS

JUDEOPHOBIA
Jew-deo-foe-bee-ah
Although there is no direct Latin or Greek word to explain the origins of this word, Judea was the ancient home of the Jews which perhaps explains the derivation of this term.

BOLSHEVIKS

BOLSHEPHOBIA
Bol-she-foe-bee-ah
Although the Bolsheviks arrived many centuries after the Greeks and Romans, the name bolshevik may originate from the Greek word *bola*, meaning to throw.

FOREIGN LANGUAGES

XENOGLOSSOPHOBIA
Zee-no-gloh-so-foe-bee-ah
The Greek words *xeno*, meaning foreigner, and *glosso*, meaning language, clarify this phobias origins.

Related Phobias:
GLOSSOPHOBIA, fear of speaking in public

GREEK TERMS OR CULTURE

HELLOPHOBIA
Hell-oh-foe-bee-ah
or
HELLENOLOGOPHOBIA
Hell-en-oh-log-o-foe-bee-ah
Hellenic is the ancient Greek language. Add to this *logo*, the Greek for speech, and the derivations of this hatred become clear.

RUSSIANS

RUSSOPHOBIA
Rus-so-foe-bee-ah
There is no Greek or Latin word to explain the origin of this term.

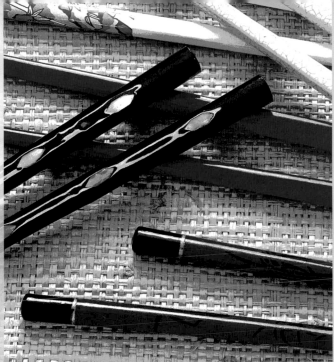

JAPANESE OR JAPANESE CULTURE

JAPANOPHOBIA
Jap-an-oh-foe-bee-ah
There is no Greek or Latin word that can trace the ancient origin for this term, however it is easy to see that takes its name from the modern word.

CHINESE OR CHINESE CULTURE

SINOPHOBIA
Sy-no-foe-bee-ah
There is no known Greek or Latin word that can trace the origins of this word.

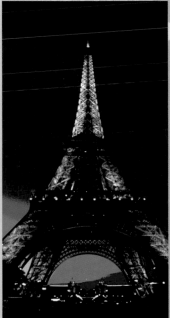

FRANCE OR FRENCH CULTURE

FRANCOPHOBIA
Fran-co-foe-bee-ah
or
GALLOPHOBIA
Gal-oh-foe-bee-ah
or
GALIPHOBIA
Gal-ee-foe-bee-ah
This strong dislike for French customs and people does not emanate from the ancient Greek or Latin languages but directly originates from the modern name France. However, the ancient Latin name for France was *gallofrom*, from which we inherit gallophobia and galiphobia.

GERMANS OR GERMAN CULTURE

GERMANOPHOBIA
Jur-man-oh-foe-bee-ah
or
TEUTOPHOBIA
Tew-toe-foe-bee-ah
While there is no direct Greek or Latin word to explain the derivation of Teutophobia, it is obviously linked to *teutonic*, which means of the German people. The Latin word for Germany was originally *Germania*, which explains the root of this tree of words.

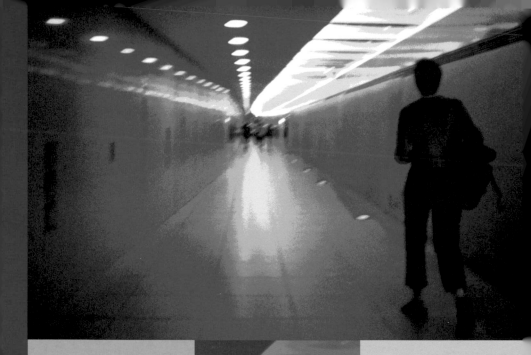

LONELINESS OR BEING BY ONESELF

EREMOPHOBIA
Air-em-oh-foe-bee-ah
or
EREMIPHOBIA
Air-em-i-foe-bee-ah
This fear of being alone or in an uninhabited place, finds its root meaning in the Greek word *eremo*, meaning solitary or hermit.

Related Phobias:
SYMBIOPHOBIA, fear of being intimate with another

BEING ALONE OR SOLITUDE

ISOLOPHOBIA
Eye-sol-oh-foe-bee-ah
This fear of one's own company finds its origins in the Latin word *soli*, which means alone and is the root of solitude.

Related Phobias:
MONOPHOBIA, fear of being alone or desolate places

FEAR OF BEING EVALUATED NEGATIVELY IN SOCIAL SITUATIONS

SOCIALPHOBIA
So-she-al-foe-bee-ah
Socio is the Latin word for relationship and provides the root meaning for this unfortunate fear.

Realted Phobias:
SOCIOPHOBIA, hatred of social situations

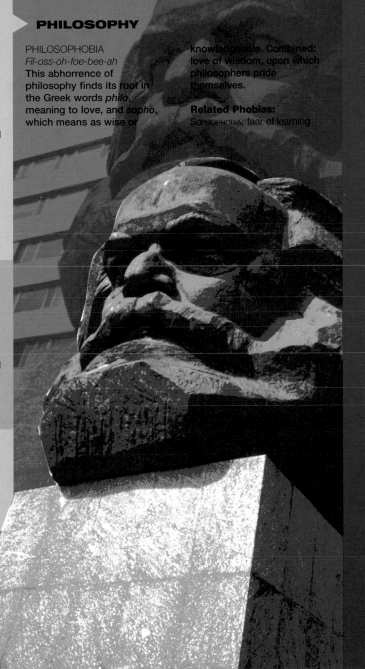

SAFETY FROM ONE'S OWN PHOBIAS

COUNTERPHOBIA
Kown-ter-foe-bee-ah
This perverse seeking out of what scares oneself is derived from the Latin prefix *counter*, meaning against.

Related Phobias:
PHOBOPHOBIA, fear of fear

DEPENDENCE ON OTHERS

SOTERIOPHOBIA
So-te-ree-oh-foe-bee-ah
The origins of this term are obscure and cannot be traced in either Latin or Greek.

BECOMING MAD

LYSSOPHOBIA
Liss-oh-foe-bee-ah
Lysso is the Greek word for madness or fury, and explains the origins of this fear of having to deal with madness, either personally or someone else's.

PHILOSOPHY

PHILOSOPHOBIA
Fil-oss-oh-foe-bee-ah
This abhorrence of philosophy finds its root in the Greek words *philo*, meaning to love, and *sopho*, which means as wise or knowledgeable. Combined: love of wisdom, upon which philosophers pride themselves.

Related Phobias:
SOPHOPHOBIA, fear of learning

IMPERFECTION

ATELOPHOBIA
At-el-oh-foe-bee-ah
This fear of not perfecting one's work or oneself originates in meaning from the Greek word *teleo*, meaning perfection.

Related Phobias:
PARALIPHOBIA, fear of neglecting one's responsibilities

RESPONSIBILITY

HYPENGYOPHOBIA
Hi-pen-jio-foe-bee-ah
or
HYPEGIAPHOBIA
Hi-per-jia-foe-bee-ah
This abhorrence for responsibility may well derive from the Latin word *hypen* meaning to bring together, as in hyphenate.

EVERYTHING

PANOPHOBIA
Pan-oh-foe-bee-ah
or
PANTOPHOBIA
Pan-toe-foe-bee-ah
or
PAMPHOBIA
Pam-foe-bee-ah
Pan and *panto* are the Greek words for all or every, which explain the origins of this nonspecific fear of everything.

Related Phobias:
POLYPHOBIA, fear of many things

HEARING GOOD NEWS
EUPHOBIA
You-foe-bee-ah
Eu is the Greek word for happy or pleasing, which gives us the origin for this fear of success and pleasure.

GAIETY

CHEROPHOBIA
Ch-air-oh-foe-bee-ah
This excessive fear of happiness or the dread that gaiety may then be followed by ill fortune derives in meaning from the Greek verb *chero*, meaning to rejoice.

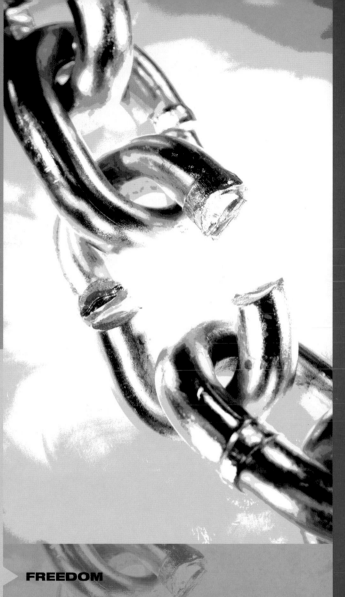

PERSONAL BODY ODOR

BROMIDROSIPHOBIA
Brom-id-row-si-foe-bee-ah
or
BROMIDROPHOBIA
Brom-id-row-foe-bee-ah
or
OSMOPHOBIA
Os-mo-foe-bee-ah
Bromo is the Greek word for stench or stink, and *id* means condition. Combined, they form a smelly condition, which provides us with the word origin of this unfortunate fear. *Osmo* is the Greek word for pungent, illuminating the root meaning of osmophobia.

THAT ONE HAS A VILE ODOR

AUTODYSOMOPHOBIA
or-toe-die-so-mo-foe-bee-ah
The Greek words *auto*, meaning self, and *dys*, meaning ill or harsh, hold some clues to this fear of personal hygiene.

Related Phobias:
OSPHRESIOPHOBIA, fear of bodily odors

FREEDOM

ELEUTHEROPHOBIA
El-you-thur-oh-foe-bee-ah
Eluthero is the Greek word for freedom, which provides the root for this term.

Related Phobias:
CLAUSTROPHOBIA, fear of being locked in a confined space

DUTY OR RESPONSIBILITY

PARALIPHOBIA
Pa-ral-ee-foe-bee-ah
Derived from the Greek word *para* meaning to protect, this phobia can relate to a fear of having responsibilities or neglecting one's responsibilities.

Related Phobias:
ATELOPHOBIA, fear of imperfection

CRITICISM

ENISSOPHOBIA
En-iss-oh-foe-bee-ah
There is no Latin or Greek word to explain the origins of this term.

WEAKNESS

ASTHENOPHOBIA
Ass-thuh-no-foe-bee-ah
This term is directly evolved from the Greek word *astheno*, meaning without strength, and literally translates as the fear of losing one's strength.

LONG WAITS

MACROPHOBIA
Mac-row-foe-bee-ah
Commonly experienced, this hatred of waiting is directly derived from the Greek word *macro*, meaning large or long.

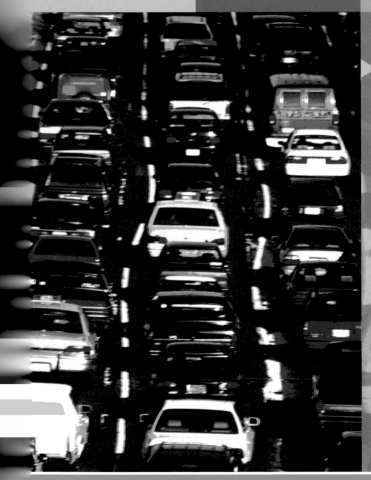

emotions

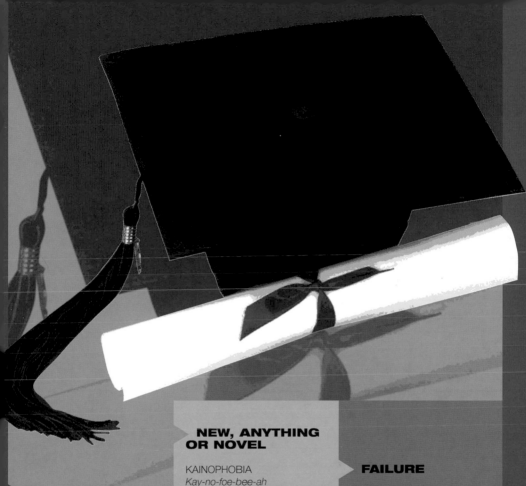

KNOWLEDGE

GNOSIOPHOBIA
No-sio-foe-bee-ah
or
EPISTEMOPHOBIA
Ep-iss-tem-o-foe-bee-ah
Gno is the Greek verb to learn or discern, while *epistemo* is the Greek verb to understand.

Related phobias:
SOPHOPHOBIA, fear of learning

NEW, ANYTHING OR NOVEL

KAINOPHOBIA
Kay-no-foe-bee-ah
or
CENOPHOBIA
Sen-oh-foe-bee-ah
or
NEOPHOBIA
Neo-foe-bee-ah
The Greek words for new are *ceno* and *neo*, which provides the base for these identical fears.

FAILURE

ATYCHIPHOBIA
At-it-chi-foe-bee-ah
or
KAKORRHAPHIOPHOBIA
Ka-kor-aff-io-foe-bee-ah
There are no Greek or Latin words that can explain the origins of atychiphobia. Kakorrhaphiophobia derives from the Greek prefix *caco*, meaning bad or unpleasant.

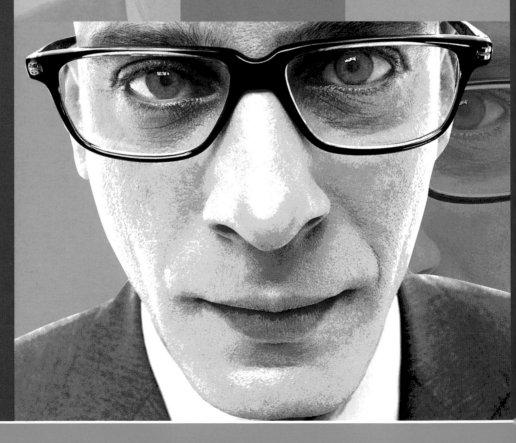

BEING SEEN OR LOOKED AT

SCOPTOPHOBIA
Skop-toe-foe-bee-ah
or
SCOPOPHOBIA
Skop-oh-foe-bee-ah
Scopo is the Greek verb to examine, explaining not only the origin of this fear of being stared at but also other contemporary words such as periscope and microscope.

Related Phobias:
EISOPTROPHOBIA, fear of looking at oneself in the mirror

RUIN

ATEPHOBIA
At-ay-foe-bee-ah
This fear of disasters such as floods, famine, or fire possibly finds its origin in the Latin prefix *ate*, meaning act, as in act of God.

Related Phobias:
THEOPHOBIA, fear of God

DEFEAT

KAKORRHAPHIOPHOBIA
Ka-kor-aff-io-foe-bee-ah
This fear of failure or dread of poor planning derives from the Greek prefix *caco*, meaning bad or unpleasant.

Related Phobias:
EUPHOBIA, fear of success

BEING TOUCHED

APHENPHOSMOPHOBIA
A-fen-fos-mo-foe-bee-ah
or
HAPHEPHOBIA
Haff-e-foe-bee-ah
or
HAPTEPHOBIA
Hap-tey-foe-bee-ah
or
CHIRAPTOPHOBIA
Chae-rap-toe-foe-bee-ah
There is no Latin or Greek word to explain the origins of aphenphosmophobia. The Greek words *chiro*, meaning hand, and *hapto*, meaning touch, clearly show how these terms were formed.

ANGER

ANGROPHOBIA
Ang-row-foe-bee-ah
or
CHOLEROPHOBIA
Kol-ero-foe-bee-ah
While angrophobia is derived from the modern word angry, cholerophobia originates in meaning from the Greek word *cholera*, meaning to discharge bile violently.

Related Phobias:
SCELEROPHOBIA, fear of wicked persons

TREMBLING

TREMOPHOBIA
Tre-mo-foe-bee-ah
This phobia finds its origin in the Latin word *tremo*, meaning to shake, from this we also obtain the modern words tremor and tremulous.

Related Phobias:
PHOBOPHOBIA, fear of fear

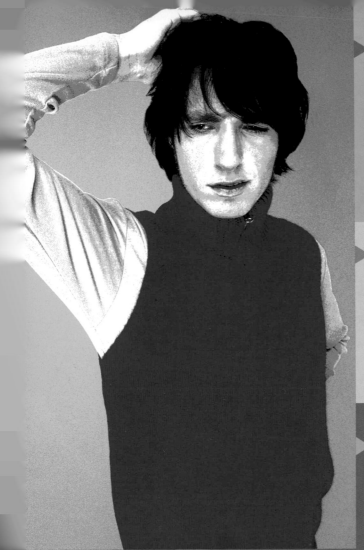

IDEAS

IDEOPHOBIA
Id-eo-foe-bee-ah
The Greek word for idea is *ideo*, which explains this dread of creativity.

Related Phobias:
PHILOSOPHOBIA, fear of philosophy

PHOBIAS

PHOBOPHOBIA
Foe-bo-foe-bee-ah
This horror of one's own fears or fear itself derives from the Greek word for fear – *phobo*.

FEELING PLEASURE

HEDONOPHOBIA
Hed-on-oh-foe-bee-ah
This repressive fear of enjoying oneself derives from the Greek word *hedonia*, meaning pleasure. From this word we also get the modern term hedonist.

Related phobias:
OENOPHOBIA, fear of wine

FORGETTING OR BEING FORGOTTEN

ATHAZAGORAPHOBIA
Ath-az-ah-gor-ah-foe-bee-ah
There are no Greek or Latin words that can help us trace the origin of this term.

EXPRESSING OPINIONS

DOXOPHOBIA
Doc-so-foe-bee-ah
Often related to a fear of being criticized, this phobia finds its root meaning in *dox*, the Greek word for opinion. From this we also derive the common terms, dogmatic and indoctrinate.

Related Phobias:
KATAGELOPHOBIA, fear of being ridiculed

BEING DIRTY

AUTOMYSOPHOBIA
or-toe-my-so-foe-bee-ah
If we combine the Greek words *auto*, meaning self, and *myso*, meaning filth, it is easy to see how we have arrived at the formation of this fear of being unclean.

MEMORIES

MNEMOPHOBIA
Nem-oh-foe-bee-ah
Mnemon is the Greek word for memory, which explains the origin of this fear of one's own past.

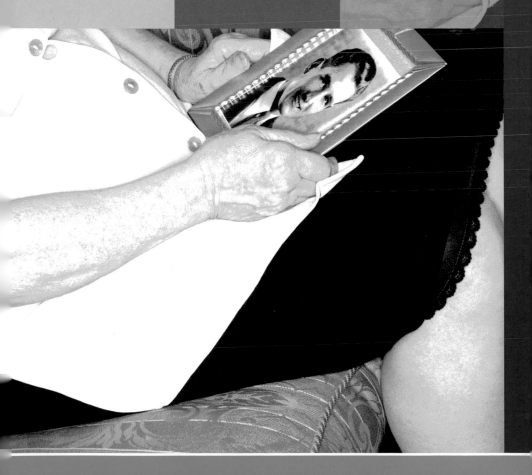

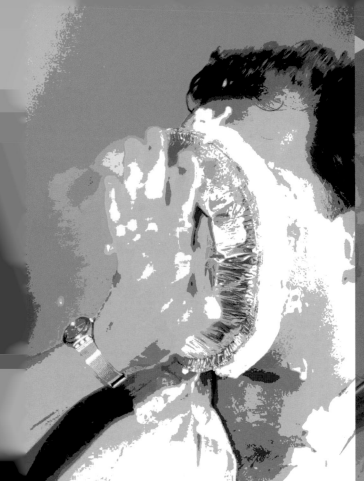

BEING RIDICULED

KATAGELOPHOBIA
Kat-a-jel-oh-foe-bee-ah
or
CATAGELOPHOBIA
Cat-a-jel-oh-foe-bee-ah
Cata is the Greek word for down or lower, which explains the origins of this fear of being put down, or having one's status lowered by others.

Related phobias:
OPTHALMOPHOBIA, fear of being stared at

JEALOUSY

ZELOPHOBIA
Zel-oh-foe-bee-ah
This fear of becoming jealous originates in meaning from the Latin word *zelo*, meaning jealous or zealous.

PROGRESS

PROSOPHOBIA
Pro-so-foe-bee-ah
This aversion to progress derives from the Latin prefix *pro*, meaning forward or in front.

MIND

PSYCHOPHOBIA
Sy-ko-foe-bee-ah
This dread of one's own mind emanates in meaning from the Greek word for mind or psyche – *psycho*. From this ancient term, we also derive such modern usages as psychology and psychopath.

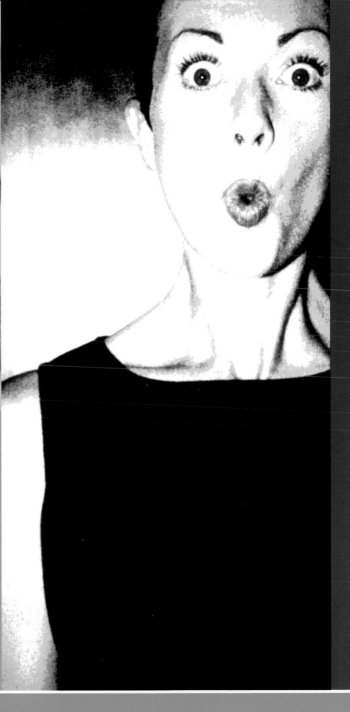

SHOCK

HORMEPHOBIA
Hor-me-foe-bee-ah
This fear of being shocked either by bad news or electrical currents, emanates from the Greek word *horm*, meaning impulse.

STAGE FRIGHT

TOPOPHOBIA
Top-oh-foe-bee-ah
This fear of stage-fright can also relate to a fear of certain places (like the stage) and originates from the Greek word *topo*, meaning place or region.

Related Phobias:
THEATROPHOBIA, fear of theaters

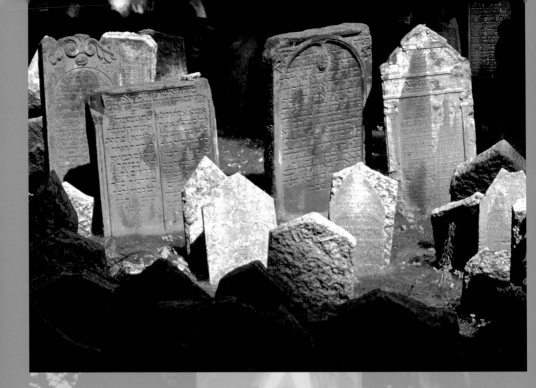

TOMBSTONES

PLACOPHOBIA
Pla-ko-foe-bee-ah
The origins of placophobia are somewhat obscure but may be derived from the Latin word *placi*, meaning calm or peace, in this case relating to a place where one finally rests. From this word we also obtain the common usage, placid.

Related Phobias:
COIMETROPHOBIA, fear of cemeteries

CEMETERIES

COIMETROPHOBIA
Coy-met-row-foe-bee-ah
Coimetro is the Greek word for sleeping room or burial place, and gives us a direct root to this fear of cemeteries.

Related Phobias:
LYGOPHOBIA, fear of dark, gloomy places

CEMETERIES OR BEING BURIED ALIVE

TAPHEPHOBIA
Taf-e-foe-bee-ah
or
TAPHOPHOBIA
Taf-o-foe-bee-ah
This popular fear can be traced in origin to the Greek word *tapho*, meaning tomb or grave, and is sometimes related to a fear of being buried alive.

Related Phobias:
NYCTOPHOBIA, fear of darkness

DEATH OR DEAD THINGS

NECROPHOBIA
Neck-row-fro-bee-ah
This dread of dead bodies derives from the Greek word *necro*, meaning death or corpse, as do other modern words such as necropolis and the morbid necrophilia.

Related Phobias:
PHASMOPHOBIA, fear of ghosts

DEATH OR DYING

THANATOPHOBIA
Than-at-oh-foe-bee-ah
This paranoid terror of dying comes from the Greek word for death – *thanato*.

THEOLOGY

THEOLOGICOPHOBIA
Thee-o-lo-gi-ko-foe-bee-ah
This distrust of religious doctrine or hatred of its sometimes obscure concepts can be traced in origin to the Greek word *theo*, which means god.

CHURCH

ECCLESIOPHOBIA
Ek-lee-see-o-foe-bee-ah
This unholy dread of churches and organized religion can be easily traced in origin to the Greek for church, *ecclesio*.

Related Phobias:
THEOPHOBIA, fear of God.

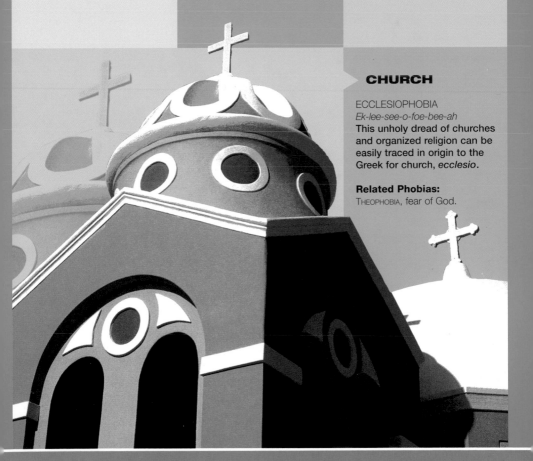

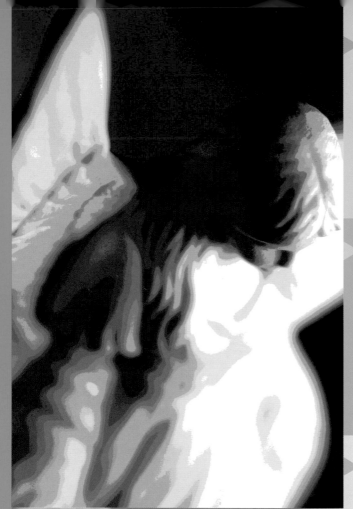

HEAVEN

OURANOPHOBIA
Ooh-ra-no-foe-bee-ah
or
URANOPHOBIA
Yu-ray-no-foe-bee-ah
Urano is the Greek word for heaven, in itself a derivation of Uranus, the mythological king of the heavens.

MATERIALISM

HYLEPHOBIA
Hi-li-foe-bee-ah
Matter or substance, as well as wood and forest are the translations from the Greek *hylo*, which commonly refers to a hatred of materialism.

Related Phobias:
AUROPHOBIA, hatred of gold and wealth

RELIGIOUS CEREMONIES

TELEOPHOBIA
Tel-ee-o-foe-bee-ah
The origins of this word are not transparent, yet we can interpret the Greek word *teleo*, meaning end or fulfilment as the root from which this term was obtained. Teleophobia may therefore, have begun as a term describing a fear of last rites and funerals.

HOLY THINGS

HAGIOPHOBIA
Haj-ee-o-foe-bee-ah
Hagio is the Greek word for holy or saint, and provides us with the root of this term.

SINNING

PECCATOPHOBIA
Pek-a-toe-foe-bee-ah
Peccato is the Latin word for
sin and gives rise to the
meaning of this term; from
this we also derive the
modern word peccadillo,
meaning misdemeanor.

COMMITTING A SIN

ENOSIOPHOBIA
Ee-nos-ee-o-foe-bee-ah
or
ENISSOPHOBIA
En-iss-o-foe-bee-ah
or
HAMARTOPHOBIA
Ham-ah-toe-foe-bee-ah
Neither enosiophobia or
enissohobia can be traced in
meaning to either Greek or
Latin words. But
hamartophobia derives from
the word *hamarto*, meaning
sin or error

SERMONS

HOMILOPHOBIA
Hom-ill-o-foe-bee-ah
Homilo is the Greek word
for assembly or meeting
and therefore provides us
with the origin of this hatred
of sermons and being
preached to.

Related Phobias:
HERESOPHOBIA, fear of deviating
from orthodox doctrine

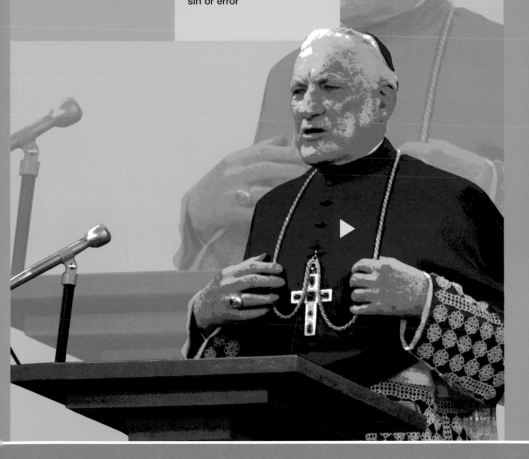

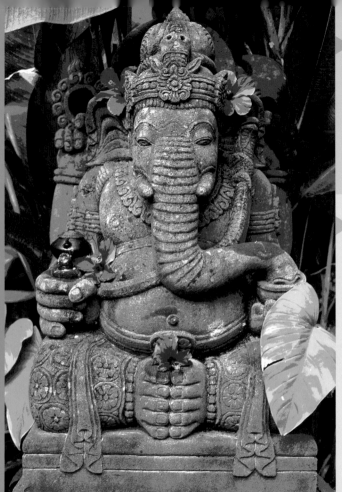

CROSSES OR THE CRUCIFIX

STAUROPHOBIA
Stor-o-foe-bee-ah
Stauro is the Greek word for cross-like or upright and provides us with the root of this term.

HELL

HADEPHOBIA
Hay-dee-foe-bee-ah
or
STYGIOPHOBIA
Sti-gee-o-foe-bee-ah
This dread of Hell or going to Hell derives in both cases from the Greek word *Hades* for the underworld, and *stygio*, meaning hate or spiteful. Historically, the ancient Greeks believed their souls would be transported to the underworld via the infernal river Styx.

GOD OR GODS

ZEUSOPHOBIA
Zee-use-o-foe-bee-ah
The undisputed king of the Gods on Mount Olympus, Zeus reigned almighty in the minds of ancient Greece. This particular fear can relate to a dread of many gods, or of a singular god.

GODS OR RELIGION

THEOPHOBIA
Thi-o-foe-bee-ah
This fear of religion emanates from the Greek word *theo*, meaning deity. From this we also derive such common usages as monotheism, theocratic and theology.

DEMONS

DEMONOPHOBIA
Dee-mon-o-foe-bee-ah
This dreaded fear derives
directly from the Greek word
demono meaning devil,
demon, or evil spirit.

Related Phobias:
BOGYPHOBIA, fear of the
Bogeyman.

SATAN

SATANOPHOBIA
Say-tan-o-foe-bee-ah
A dread of the devil, satanists
or being demonically
possessed, this term finds its
origin in the Greek and Hebrew
word *satan*, meaning
adversary or devil.

CHALLENGES TO OR RADICAL DEVIATION FROM OFFICIAL DOCTRINE

HERESYPHOBIA
Heh-re-si-foe-bee-ah
or
HEREIOPHOBIA
Heh-ree-o-foe-bee-ah
The origins of this term are
derived from the Latin word
her, meaning to stick to, as in
social, personal beliefs. From
this we also obtain
contemporary words like
adhere and heresy.

PRIESTS OR SACRED THINGS

HIEROPHOBIA
He-row-foe-bee-ah
This fear of clergymen and
objects of holy value can be
directly traced in meaning to
the Greek word *hiero*, meaning
sacred.

Related Phobias:
ECCLESIOPHOBIA, fear
of church

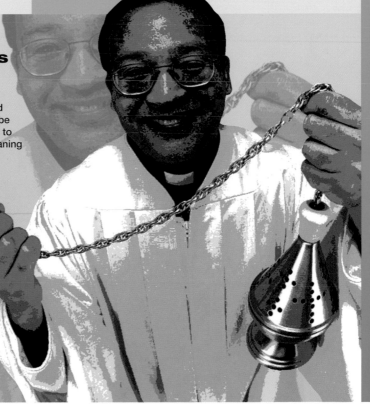

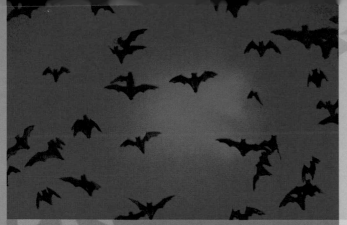

BATS

VESPERTILIOPHOBIA
Ves-per-til-ee-o-foe-bee-ah
Vespertilio is the Latin for bat, in itself a derivative of *vesper*, the Latin word for evening or of the night.

SPECTERS

SPECTROPHOBIA
Sp-ek-tro-foe-bee-ah
Spec is the Latin word for spectacle or sight. Phobics of this disorder may fear looking in a mirror for dread of seeing something other than their own reflection.

DREAMS

ONEIROPHOBIA
Oh-nee-row-foe-bee-ah
Oneiro is the Greek verb to dream and therefore provides us with a clear explanation of this terms origin.

Related Phobias:
ONEIROGMOPHOBIA, fear of wet dreams.

GHOSTS

PHASMOPHOBIA
Fas-mo-foe-bee-ah
This common fear, usually experienced by children, can be traced in meaning to the Greek word *phasmato*, meaning ghost. More commonly used words such as phantasmagoria also evolve from the latter.

SPIRITS

PNEUMATOPHOBIA
Nu-mat-o-foe-bee-ah
This fear of incorporeal forms finds its root in the Greek word *pneumato*, meaning presence or spirit.

Related Phobias:
DEMONOPHOBIA, fear of evil spirits

MYTHS OR STORIES OR FALSE STATEMENTS

MYTHOPHOBIA
My-tho-foe-bee-ah
This excessive fear of being told a story not based in reality, or the fear of hearing something which is not entirely correct, aptly finds its origin in the Greek word *mytho*, meaning legend or myth.

BOGEYMAN OR BOGIES

BOGYPHOBIA
Bo-gee-foe-bee-ah
There is no Greek or Latin word that can help us trace the origin of this word.

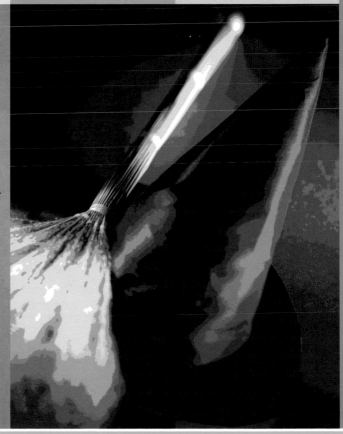

WITCHES AND WITCHCRAFT

WICCAPHOBIA
Wik-ka-foe-be-ah
Although there are no Greek or Roman words that can identify this term, *wicca* is an age-old pagan religion predating the Romans, and was first practiced by the druids in England. It is from this denomination that we extract this fear of Witchcraft.

BLOOD

HEMOPHOBIA
Hem-o-foe-bee-ah
or
HEMAPHOBIA
Hem-a-foe-bee-ah
or
HEMATOPHOBIA
Hem-at-o-foe-bee-ah
The Greek word for blood is *hem*, which gives us the both the direct origin of this word, as well as a number of contemporary medical terms such as hemophiliac.

HEART

CARDIOPHOBIA
Car-dee-o-foe-bee-ah
This dreaded fear of heart attacks or heart disease takes its meaning from the Greek word *cardio*, meaning heart. Contemporary medical terms such as cardiac and cardiography (measuring of the heart) also stem from this root.

HANDS

CHIROPHOBIA
Ch-aye-o-foe-bee-ah
The Greek word *chiro* means hand and is also used to define chirography (handwriting) and chiromancy (palmistry).

LEFT-HANDED

SINISTROPHOBIA
Sin-iss-tro-foe-bee-ah
This fear can literally be traced to the Latin term *sinistro*, which means left-handed.

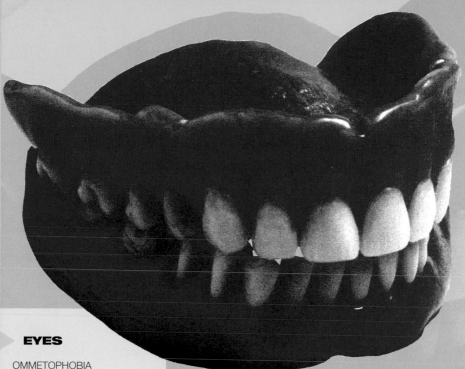

EYES

OMMETOPHOBIA
Om-met-a-foe-bee-ah
or
OMMATOPHOBIA
Omm-mat-o-foe-bee-ah
This excessive fear of eyes emanates from the Greek word *ommat*, meaning eye.

TEETH

ODONTOPHOBIA
O-don-toe-foe-bee-ah
Odonto is the Greek for of the tooth. The Latin word for tooth is *dent*, which gives us contemporary words such as dentistry, dental, and dentist.

Related Phobias:
DENTAOPHOBIA, fear of dentists

OPENING ONES EYES

OPTOPHOBIA
Op-toe-foe-bee-ah
Opticois, the Greek word for sight, gives direct rise to this fear of opening ones eyes.

GETTING WRINKLES

RHYTIPHOBIA
Rye-tee-foe-bee-ah
This excessive fear of getting wrinkles finds its origin in the Greek word *rhytid*, literally meaning wrinkle

Related Phobias:
GERONTOPHOBIA, fear of growing old

CHINS

GENIOPHOBIA
Jen-ee-o-foe-bee-ah
The origins of the *gen-* prefix are obscure, but it may originate from the old Germanic or English word *cin(n)* meaning chin.

Related Phobias:
POGONOPHOBIA, fear of beards

KNEES

GENUPHOBIA
Jen-yew-foe-bee-ah
This fear of knees or servility (having to get down on ones knee) takes its definition from the Greek word *genu*, meaning knee.

Related Phobias:
TYRANNOPHOBIA, fear of tyrants

RECTUM

PROCTOPHOBIA
Prok-toe-foe-bee-ah
or
RECTOPHOBIA
Rek-toe-foe-bee-ah
The Latin and Greek words *procto* and *recto*, both meaning anus, give us the direct root of these anal phobias.

FATIGUE

KOPOPHOBIA
Kop-o-foe-bee-ah
Kopo is the Greek word for weariness or exhaustion and therefore provides us with the origin of this term.

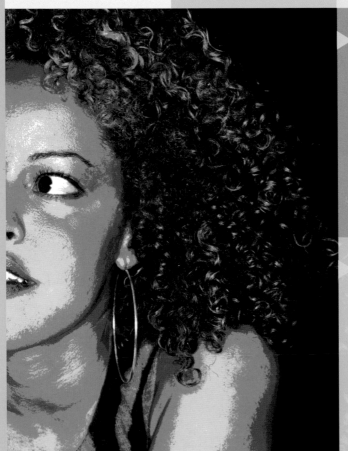

HAIR

CHAETOPHOBIA
Ky-toe-foe-bee-ah
This general abhorrence toward hair is derived from the Greek word *chaeto*, meaning long, flowing hair.

Related Phobias:
PELADOPHOBIA, fear of going bald or baldness

HAIR DISEASE

TRICHOPATHOPHOBIA
Try-ko-pa-tho-foe-bee-ah
This fear of catching a hair disorder is a combination of the Greek words *tricho*, meaning hair, and *patho*, which translates as suffering.

Related Phobias:
HYPERTRICHOPHOBIA, fear of excessively bad hair diseases

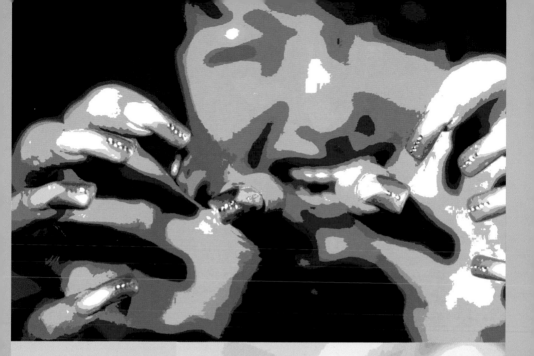

FECAL MATTER

COPROPHOBIA
Kop-row-foe-bee-ah
or
SCATOPHOBIA
Sca-toe-foe-bee-ah
Both these phobias take their names from the Greek words *copro* and *scato*, meaning filth or excrement.

Related phobias:
MYSOPHOBIA, fear of being contaminated by dirt

SCRATCHES OR BEING SCRATCHED

AMYCHIPHOBIA
A-mich-e-foe-bee-ah

Amycho is the Greek verb to scratch and provides us with the direct origin of this particular fear.

Related Phobias:
ACARAPHOBIA, fear of itching

THINGS TO THE LEFT SIDE OF THE BODY

LEVOPHOBIA
Lev-o-foe-bee-ah
This excessive fear of things on the left side of the body emanates in meaning from the Latin *levo*, meaning left.

THINGS TO THE RIGHT SIDE OF THE BODY

DEXTROPHOBIA
Dex-tro-foe-bee-ah
Dextro, the Latin word for right or the right side, leads us to this fear of things on the right side.

CHEST PAIN

ANGINOPHOBIA
An-jye-no-foe-bee-ah
This fear of heartburn or angina takes its name from the Greek word *angio*, meaning blood vessel.

Related Phobias:
CARDIOPHOBIA, fear of heart attack

EATING OR SWALLOWING

PHAGOPHOBIA
Fag-oh-foe-bee-ah
This fear of eating finds its meaning in the Greek verb *phago* meaning to consume.

BEING CHOKED OR SMOTHERED

PNIGOPHOBIA
Nig-o-foe-bee-ah
or
PNIGEROPHOBIA
Nig-er-o-foe-bee-ah
This common fear derives in meaning from the Greek verb to choke – *pnigo*. Sufferers of this phobia are more concerned with choking in their sleep than when awake.

Related phobias:
ONEIROPHOBIA, fear of bad dreams

PAIN

ALGOPHOBIA
Al-gee-foe-bee-ah
or
PONOPHOBIA
Pon-o-foe-bee-ah
or
ODYNOPHOBIA
Oh-din-o-foe-bee-ah
or
ODYNEPHOBIA
Oh-din-e-foe-bee-ah
All these variants of the fear of pain find their derivation in the Greek words *algo*, *pono*, and *odyno* literally meaning pain.

Related Phobias:
ERGOPHOBIA, fear of work

LAUGHTER

GELIOPHOBIA
Jel-ee-o-foe-bee-ah
This excessive fear derives in origin from the Greek word *gelato* meaning laughter.

Related Phobias:
CHEROPHOBIA, fear of happiness.

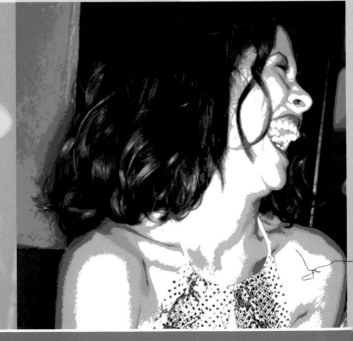

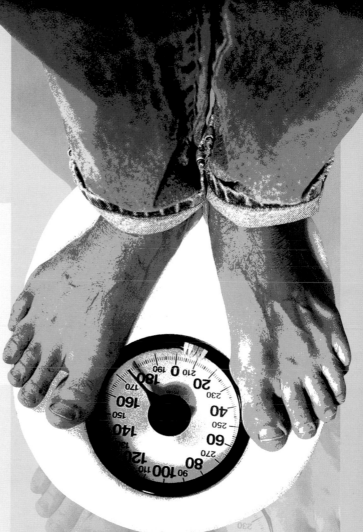

FAINTING

ASTHENOPHOBIA
Ass-thuh-no-foe-bee-ah
This term directly evolved from the Greek word *astheno*, meaning without strength and literally translates as the fear of losing one's strength (to remain upright).

STOOPING

KYPHOPHOBIA
Ky-foe-foe-bee-ah
Often related to a fear of falling over or damaging one's back by changing posture, this fear emanates from the Greek word *kypho*, meaning hunchbacked or bent.

CHILDBIRTH

MALEUSIOPHOBIA
Ma-lee-us-e-o-foe-bee-ah
or
TOCOPHOBIA
Toh-ko-foe-bee-ah
or
PARTURIPHOBIA
Pa-ch-ree-foe-bee-ah
or
LOCKIOPHOBIA
Lo-kee-o-foe-bee-ah
Of all these similar phobias, only tocophobia and parturiphobia can be traced: the Greek word *toco* means childbirth or delivery, as does the Latin word *para*, which gives us parturiphobia.

GAINING WEIGHT

OBESOPHOBIA
Oh-bee-so-foe-bee-ah
or
POCRESCOPHOBIA
Po-kri-sko-foe-bee-ah

These identical fears derive in meaning from the Latin words *obeso* and *pocre*, meaning obese and pig.

Related Phobias:
CATAGELOPHOBIA, fear of being laughed at

SPEAKING

LALIOPHOBIA
La-lee-oh-foe-bee-ah
or
LALOPHOBIA
La-lo-foe-bee-ah
This fear of stuttering or
babbling finds its origin in the
Greek word *lalio* – to chatter or
to babble.

TRYING TO SPEAK

GLOSSOPHOBIA
Gl-oss-oh-foe-bee-ah
Often associated with people
suffering from a speech
impediment, this phobia finds
its origin in the Greek word
glosso, which means tongue
or speech.

STUTTERING

PSELLISMOPHOBIA
Se-li-smo-foe-bee-ah
Psellismo, the Greek word for
stuttering, explains the root
meaning of this term.

Related Phobias:
KATAGELOPHOBIA, fear of
being ridiculed

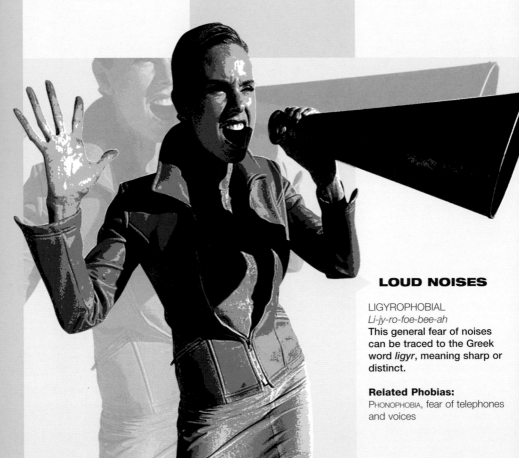

LOUD NOISES

LIGYROPHOBIAL
Li-jy-ro-foe-bee-ah
This general fear of noises
can be traced to the Greek
word *ligyr*, meaning sharp or
distinct.

Related Phobias:
PHONOPHOBIA, fear of telephones
and voices

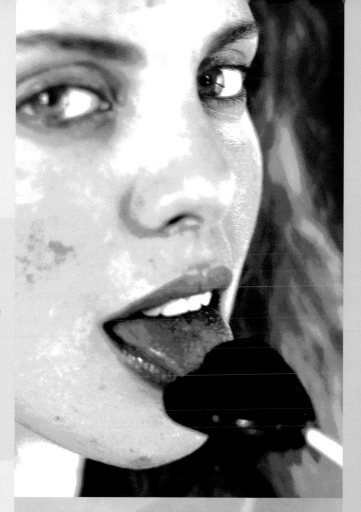

ITCHING

ACAROPHOBIA
Ak-a-ro-foe-bee-ah
Acaro is the Greek word for tiny spider or mite, but can also refer to itching.

Related Phobias:
SCABIOPHOBIA, fear of scabies

URINE OR URINATING

URINOPHOBIA
Ur-eye-no-foe-bee-ah
This fear of urinating in public places, or not being able to urinate at all, originates from the Latin word for water, wet or urine – *urino*.

Related Phobias:
DISHABILLOPHOBIA, fear of undressing in front of someone

PAINFUL BOWEL MOVEMENTS

DEFECALOESIOPHOBIA
Def-ek-al-o-esi-o-foe-bee-ah
This uncomfortable anxiety stems from the Greek word *feco* meaning fecal matter.

Related Phobias:
COPROPHOBIA, fear of feces

TASTE

GEUMAPHOBIA
Jum-a-foe-bee-ah
or
GEUMOPHOBIA
Jum-o-foe-bee-ah

Derived from the Greek word *geus*, meaning taste, this fear can relate to losing one's sense of taste or to certain tastes that may be abhorrent to the individual.

Related Phobias:
CIBOPHOBIA, fear of particular foodstuffs

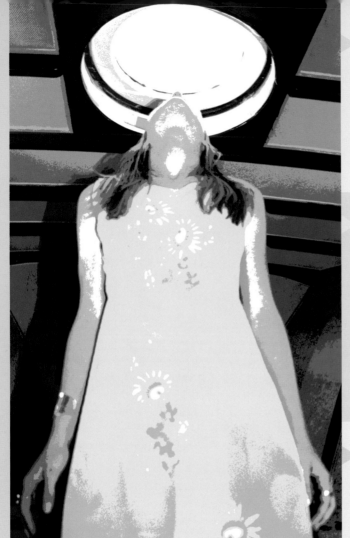

VOMITING

EMETOPHOBIA
Em-et-o-foe-bee-ah
Emeto, the Greek verb to vomit, neatly explains the origins of this common phobia.

Related Phobias:
PNIGEROPHOBIA, fear of choking

DOUBLE VISION

DIPLOPHOBIA
Dip-lo-foe-bee-ah
The Greek word *diplo*, or double, gives us the word origin of this fear.

Related Phobias:
OMMETOPHOBIA, fear of eyes

SLEEP

SOMIPHOBIA
Som-ni-foe-bee-ah
This fear of sleeping derives its meaning from the Latin verb to sleep – *somno*. From this we also obtain the contemporary term, insomnia.

Related Phobias:
CLINOPHOBIA, fear of going to bed

LOOKING UP

ANABLEPHOBIA
An-ab-lee-foe-bee-ah
This term can be traced directly to the Greek verb *anablepo*, meaning to look up. Sufferers of this phobia often experience panic attacks or dizziness when looking up at buildings or mountains.

Related Phobias:
BATOPHOBIA, fear of high buildings

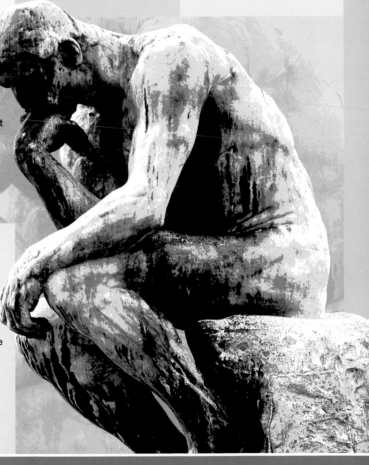

INABILITY TO STAND

BASIPHOBIA
Ba-si-foe-bee-ah
This destabilizing anxiety finds its root in the Greek word *basi*, meaning foundation or ground.

Related Phobias:
BASOSTASOPHOBIA, fear of collapsing

STANDING UPRIGHT

STASIPHOBIA
Stay-si-foe-bee-ah
or
STASIBASIPHOBIA
Stay-si-bas-oh-foe-bee-ah
The debilitating belief that one cannot stand up or walk finds its origin in the Greek words *stasi*, meaning fixed or solid, and *bas*, which means step.

SITTING

CATHISOPHOBIA
Ka-thi-so-foe-bee-ah
or
THAASOPHOBIA
Th-ah-so-foe-bee-ah
Kathiso, the Greek verb to sit, explains the seat of this hatred of sitting down. However, thaasophobia, which relates to a fear of being bored and an inability to sit still, cannot be traced to any Greek or Latin word.

THINKING

PHRONEMOPHOBIA
Fro-nem-o-foe-bee-ah
This dread of thinking derives in meaning from the Greek word *phront*, meaning thought or attention.

Related Phobias:
SOPHOPHOBIA, fear of learning

SLEEP OR BEING HYPNOTIZED

HYPNOPHOBIA
Hip-no-foe-bee-ah
Hypnos, the Greek god of dreams, taken in turn from the Greek word *hypno*, meaning sleep, explains the origin of this fearful anxiety.

Related Phobias:
WICCAPHOBIA, fear of witches or magic

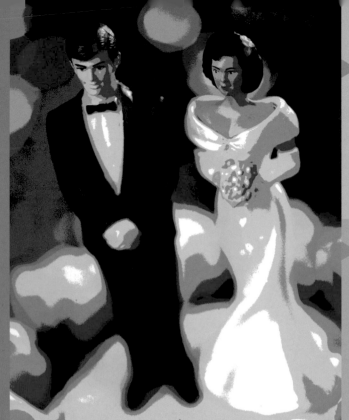

FALLING OR BEING IN LOVE

PHILOPHOBIA
Fi-lem-ah-foe-bee-ah
The derivation of this fear comes from the Greek word for love – *phile*.

COITUS

COITOPHOBIA
Coy-to-foe-bee-ah
This abnormal fear of sexual intercourse finds its root meaning in the Latin word *coition*, meaning to go.

Related Phobias:
SYMBIOPHOBIA, fear of intimacy with another

MARRIAGE

GAMOPHOBIA
Gam-o-foe-bee-ah
This common fear derives in meaning from the Greek word *gamo*, meaning marriage or union, and gives us modern suffixes such as monogamy and polygamy.

Related Phobias:
EREMOPHOBIA, fear of loneliness

FEMALE GENITALIA

EUROTOPHOBIA
Your-o-toe-foe-bee-ah
or
COLPOPHOBIA
Col-po-foe-bee-ah
There is no direct Latin or Greek word for eurotophobia. The Greek word *colpo*, meaning hollow or vagina, gives us the obvious root of this fear of female genitals.

LOVEPLAY

MALAXOPHOBIA
Mal-ax-oh-foe-bee-ah
or
SARMASSOPHOBIA
Sar-mass-oh-foe-bee-ah
Malaxo, the Greek verb to knead or stroke explains the origin of this word. The Greek for flesh is *sarx*, and *massein* is massage: combined, they form the second phobia.

STAYING SINGLE

ANUPTAPHOBIA
An-up-ta-foe-bee-ah
Often associated with the fear of growing old alone, there is no Greek or Latin word that can help us trace the origin of this word.

Related Phobias:
MONOPHOBIA, fear of being alone

SEXUAL LOVE

Erotophobia
IR-OT-OH-FOE-BEE-AH
This fear of love-making takes its meaning from Eros, the Greek god of passion and *ero*, the Greek verb to love.

SEX

GENOPHOBIA
Gen-oh-foe-bee-ah
Geno is the Greek word for race or kind, and directly pertains to sexual matters. This phobia is not gender-specific and relates to an aversion to sexual intercourse with either males or females.

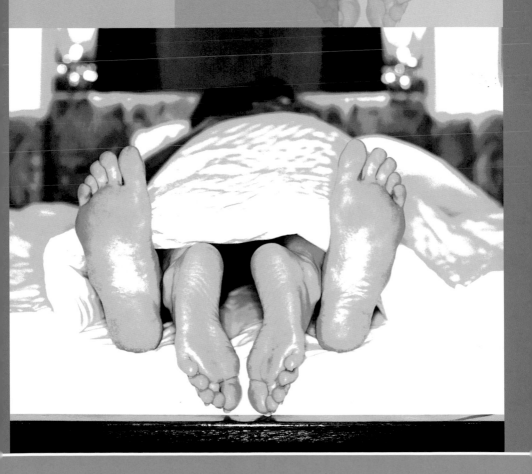

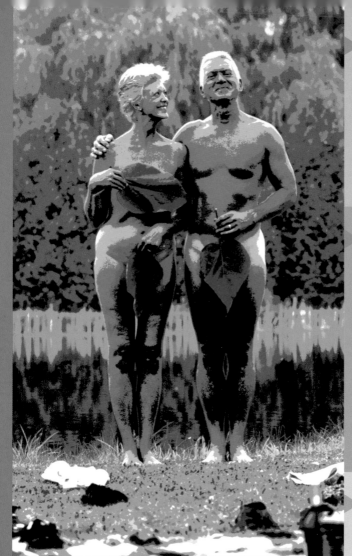

WET DREAMS

ONEIROGMOPHOBIA
Oh-nee-rog-mo-foe-bee-ah
Oneiro, the Greek verb to
dream, identifies this word.

Related Phobias:
ONEIROPHOBIA, fear of dreams and
what they might signify

SEXUAL ABUSE

AGRAPHOBIA
Ag-ra-foe-bee-ah
or
CONTRELTOPHOBIA
Con-trel-toe-foe-bee-ah
This terrible fear of sexual
abuse comes from *agriis*,
the Greek word for savage.
The seond variation of this
phobia comes from the word
contra, meaning against
or opposed to – as in
contraband or contravene.

Related Phobias:
ALGOPHOBIA, fear of pain

SEXUAL
PERVERSION

PARAPHOBIA
Pa-ra-foe-bee-ah
This dread of shaming oneself
with sexual misconduct
derives from the Greek
word *para*, meaning
wrong or abnormal.

Related Phobias:
PORNOPHOBIA, fear or aversion
to pornography

NUDITY

GYMNOPHOBIA
Jim-no-foe-bee-ah
or
NUDOPHOBIA
New-doh-foe-bee-ah

This fear of being undressed
directly relates to the Greek
words *gymno* and *nudo*, both
meaning naked.

BEAUTIFUL WOMEN

CALIGYNEPHOBIA
Kal-i-jin-ay-foe-bee-ah
Stemming from the Greek word for beautiful – *calli* – this fear of stunning women has another variation; Venusophobia, finding its root in the Ancient Greek goddess of love and beauty, Venus.

Related Phobias:
TERATOPHOBIA, fear of ugliness or malformation

VENEREAL DISEASE OR PROSTITUTES

CYPRIDOPHOBIA
Sip-rid-oh-foe-bee-ah
or
CYPRIPHOBIA
Sip-ree-foe-bee-ah
or
CYPRINOPHOBIA
Sip-rin-oh-foe-bee-ah
The excessive fear of catching sexual diseases, or contact with a prostitute, these identical phobias find their origins in the Greek word *cyprid*, meaning a lewd or licentious woman, or Kypris, meaning Venus, the goddess of love.

Related Phobias:
LUIPHOBIA, fear of catching syphilis

KISSING

PHILEMAPHOBIA
Fi-lem-ah-foe-bee-ah
or
PHILEMATOPHOBIA
Fil-em-at-oh-foe-bee-ah

The Greek word for love is *phile*, which explains the origin of this fear of kissing.

Related Phobias:
HALITOPHOBIA, fear of bad breath.

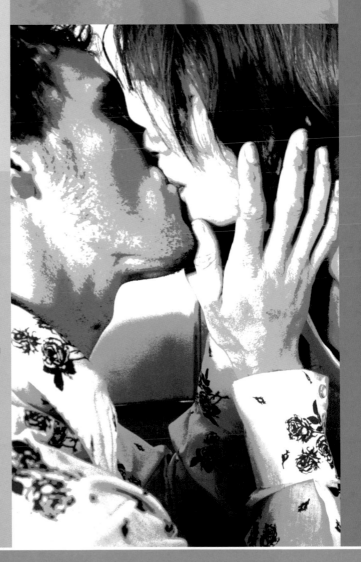

HOMOSEXUALITY OR BECOMING HOMOSEXUAL

HOMOPHOBIA
Hom-oh-foe-bee-ah
Homo is the Latin word for man, which explains the origins of this word.

PENIS

PHALLOPHOBIA
Fal-o-foe-bee-ah
The Greek word *phallus*, meaning penis, explains the meaning of this fear of the male sexual organ.

ERECTION, LOSING AN

MEDOMALACUPHOBIA
Med-o-mal-a-cue-foe-bee-ah
The origins for this word are unknown and no direct Latin or Greek link can be traced.

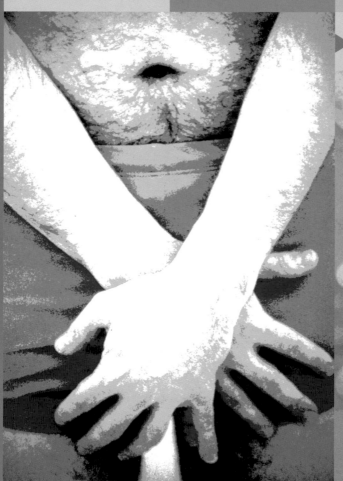

UNDRESSING IN FRONT OF SOMEONE

DISHABILLOPHOBIA
Dis-hab-ill-o-foe-bee-ah
Adysois is the Greek verb to undress, while *habili* means clothing. Together, they neatly explain the origins of this term.

Related Phobias:
CATOPTROPHOBIA, fear of seeing oneself in a mirror

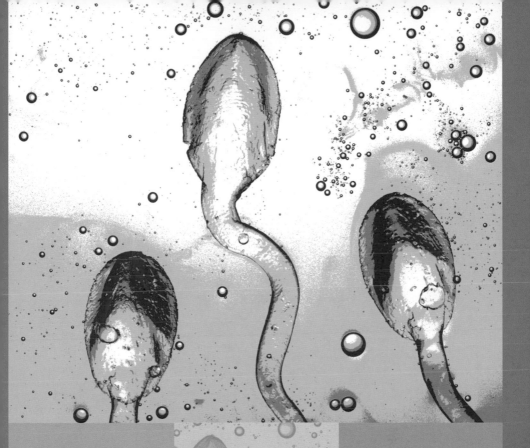

SEEING, THINKING ABOUT OR HAVING AN ERECT PENIS

ITHYPHALLOPHOBIA
Ith-ee-fal-o-foe-bee-ah
The Greek word *ithy* means straight, alludes indirectly to the erect organ.

Related Phobias:
ENISSOPHOBIA, fear of committing a sin

SEMEN

SPERMATOPHOBIA
Spur-mat-oh-foe-bee-ah
or
SPERMOPHOBIA
Spur-ma-foe-bee-ah
**This unfortunate anxiety over one's own semen is derived from the Latin word *spermo*, meaning seed.
It can also relate to a general fear of germs.**

Related Phobias:
PEDOPHOBIA, fear of children

LOSING ONE'S VIRGINITY

PRIMEISODOPHOBIA
Pri-my-sod-oh-foe-bee-ah
This rather tragic fear cannot be specifically traced to any Latin or Greek word.

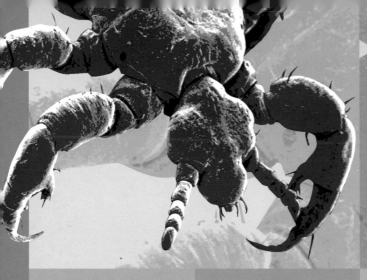

LICE

PEDICULOPHOBIA
Ped-ik-ulo-foe-bee-ah
or
PTHIRIOPHOBIA
Thi-ri-o-foe-bee-ah
This dread of being infested with lice finds its origin in the Latin word *pediculo*, meaning lice. There is, however, no Greek or Latin word that can help us explain where the term pthiriophobia emanates from.

Related Phobias:
MICROPHOBIA, fear of small things

DISEASE

NOSOPHOBIA
No-so-foe-bee-ah
or
NOSEMAPHOBIA
No-sem-a-foe-bee-ah
This exaggerated fear of catching a disease takes its name from *noso*, the Greek word for disease.

RECTAL DISEASE

RECTOPHOBIA
Rek-toe-foe-bee-ah
This extreme fear of experiencing rectal pain finds its origin in the Latin word *recto*, meaning straight or direct, as in the straight intestine that ends in the anus.

DISEASE, A DEFINITE

MONOPATHOPHOBIA
Mon-o-pa-tho-foe-bee-ah
This phobia finds its roots in the Greek word *patho* meaning disease, add to this the Greek word *mono* meaning single and it gives us a fear of a specific disease.

KIDNEY DISEASE

ALBUMINUROPHOBIA
Al-bum-in-your-o-foe-bee-ah
This fear of finding albumin in one's urine, which would suggest a problem with the kidneys, finds its root origin in the Latin word *albumino*, meaning white.

Related Phobias:
URINOPHOBIA, fear of urinating

DISEASE AND SUFFERING

PANTHOPHOBIA
Pa-tho-foe-bee-ah
Patho is the Greek word for disease or suffering, providing us with the origin of this dread of catching any kind of disease.

Related Phobias:
ALGOPHOBIA, fear of pain

BRAIN DISEASE

MENINGITOPHOBIA
Men-in-ji-toe-foe-bee-ah
This cerebral fear of brain disease takes its origin from the Greek word for membranes surrounding the brain – *meningo*.

Related Phobias:
GERASCOPHOBIA, fear of growing old

SKIN DISEASE

DERMATOSIOPHOBIA
Dur-mat-o-si-o-foe-bee-ah
The Greek word *dermato*, meaning skin is the derivation of this fear of the discomfort caused by a skin disease, and a fear of catching one.

SKIN LESIONS

DERMATOPHOBIA
Dur-mat-o-foe-bee-ah
Being scared of having lesions or cracks on one's skin derives in meaning from the Greek word *dermato*, meaning skin.

TETANUS OR LOCKJAW

TETANOPHOBIA
Tet-an-o-foe-bee-ah
Tetano is the Greek word for muscle spasm or tension, which explains the origin of this phobia.

NOSEBLEEDS

EPISTAXIOPHOBIA
Ep-iss-tax-io-foe-bee-ah
There are no Greek or Latin words that can help us identify where this term emanates from.

Related Phobias:
HEMOPHOBIA, fear of blood

CANCER

CANCEROPHOBIA
Can-sur-o-foe-bee-ah
or
CARCINOPHOBIA
Car-sin-o-foe-bee-ah
This dread of developing cancer can be traced in origin to the same word in Latin *cancer* meaning malignant.

Related Phobias:
TOXIPHOBIA, fear of being poisoned.

SCABIES

SCABIPHOBIA
Ska-bee-foe-bee-ah
The fear of catching this irritable condition, or the seven-year itch, derives in meaning from the Latin word *scabio*, meaning literally rough or itchy.

FEVER

FEBRIPHOBIA
Feb-ri-foe-bee-ah
or
FIDRIPHOBIA
Fid-ri-foe-bee-ah
or
PYREXIOPHOBIA
Pie-rex-e-o-foe-bee-ah
Febri, the Latin word for fever, directly explains the root origin of the term febriphobia. Pyrexiophobia takes its name from the Greek word *pyro*, which translates as heat or fire.

RABIES

CYNOPHOBIA
Si-no-foe-bee-ah
or
KYNOPHOBIA
Kin-o-foe-bee-ah
or
HYDROPHOBIA
Hi-dro-foe-bee-ah
These variations of a fear of dogs or rabies are all derived in meaning from Greek words *cyno*, meaning dog, and *hydro*, meaning water. Sufferers of rabies cannot drink water, which therefore explains the formation of the word hydrophobia.

DIABETES

DIABETOPHOBIAS
Die-ah-bet-o-foe-bee-ah
This fear of becoming diabetic cannot be traced in meaning to any Greek or Latin word.

Related Phobias:
KOPOPHOBIA, fear of fatigue

MUSCULAR UNCOORDINATION (ATAXIA)

ATAXIAPHOBIA
A-tax-ee-a-foe-bee-ah
The Greek word *ataxia*, meaning disorder, provides us with the origin of this term.

DOUBLE VISION

DIPLOPHOBIA
Dip-lo-foe-bee-ah
The Greek word *diplo* meaning double gives us the word origin of this fear.

Related Phobias:
OMMETOPHOBIA, fear of eyes

CONTRACTING POLIOMYELITIS

POLIOSOPHOBIA
Po-lee-o-so-foe-bee-ah
This fear derives in name from the Greek word *polio*, meaning gray matter, as in the brain or nervous system.

Related Phobias:
MENINGITOPHOBIA, fear of brain disease

SYPHILIS (LUES)

LUIPHOBIA
Lew-ee-foe-bee-ah
or
SYPHILOPHOBIA
Sif-il-o-foe-bee-ah
These identical fears directly derive from the Latin words *lue*, meaning plague, and *syphil*, meaning the French disease.

Related Phobias:
CYPRIPHOBIA, fear of catching a sexually transmitted disease

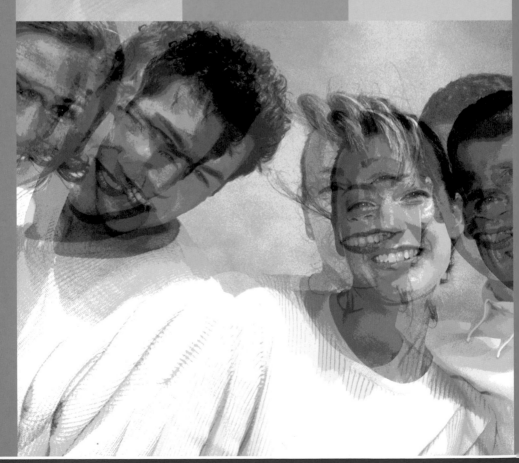

LEPROSY

LEPROPHOBIA
Lep-row-foe-bee-ah
Lepros, the Greek word for scabby or scaly, provides us with the direct word origin of this unlikely phobia.

Related Phobias:
DERMATOPHOBIA, fear of skin lesions

GROWING OLD

GERASCOPHOBIA
Jer-ass-coe-foe-bee-ah
or
GERONTOPHOBIA
Jer-on-toe-foe-bee-ah
This common fear of being left alone in old age directly derives from the Greek word *geronto*, meaning old man or old age.

CONSTIPATION

COPRASTASOPHOBIA
Cop-ra-sta-so-foe-bee-ah
The Greek words *copra*, meaning filth, and *stato*, meaning fixed or immobile, provide us with easy clues as to how this unfortunate term forms its meaning.

Related Phobias:
COPROPHOBIA, fear of feces

CHOLERA

CHOROPHOBIA
Kor-o-foe-bee-ah
Aptly, this term takes its name from the Greek word *cholo*, meaning bile.

Related Phobias:
EMETOPHOBIA, fear of vomiting

SWALLOWING AIR

AEROPHOBIA
Air-oh-foe-bee-ah
This debilitating fear finds its direct word origin in the Greek word *aero*, meaning air.

ANGINA

ANGINOPHOBIA
An-ji-no-foe-bee-ah
This fear of heartburn or angina takes its name from the Greek word *angio*, meaning blood vessel.

Related Phobias:
PNIGOPHOBIA, fear of choking

BEING INFESTED WITH WORMS

HELMINTHOPHOBIA
Hel-min-tho-foe-bee-ah
or
SCOLECIPHOBIA
Sko-lek-ee-foe-bee-ah
These identical fears find their origins in the Greek words for worm – *helmintho* and *scoleco*.

Related Phobias:
HERPETOPHOBIA, fear of creepy crawlies

JOINT IMMOBILITY

ANKYLOPHOBIA
An-kil-o-foe-bee-ah
This fear of immobility derives its root meaning from the Greek word *ankylo*, meaning stiff, crooked or unmovable.

Related phobias:
THAASOPHOBIA, fear of standing still

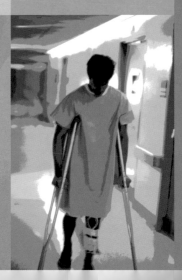

GOING TO THE DOCTORS

IATROPHOBIA
Eye-at-row-foe-bee-ah
This common dread originates in meaning from the Greek word for physician or doctor – *iatro*.

Related Phobias:
ALGOPHOBIA, fear of pain

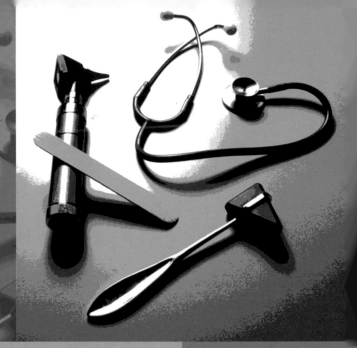

MEDICINE PRESCRIBED BY A DOCTOR

OPIOPHOBIA
Op-ee-o-foe-bee-ah

The Greek word for plant extracts (from which we obtain medicine) is *opio*, which provides us with the derivation of this phobia.

Related Phobias:
BOTANOPHOBIA, fear of plants

INJURY

TRAUMATOPHOBIA
Tr-or-ma-to-foe-bee-ah
Traumato is the Greek word for injury or wound.

Related Phobias:
PONOPHOBIA, fear of pain

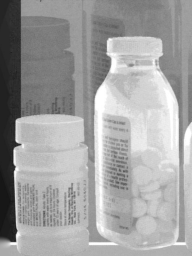

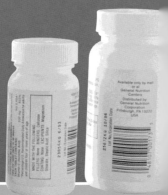

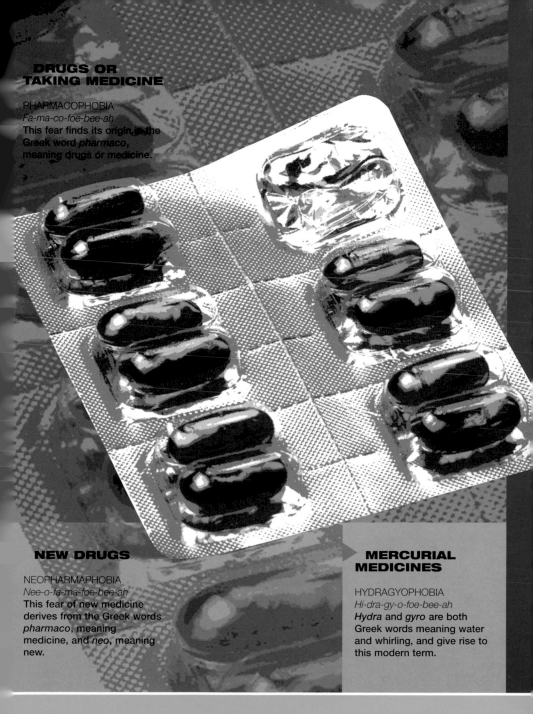

DRUGS OR TAKING MEDICINE

PHARMACOPHOBIA
Fa-ma-co-foe-bee-ah
This fear finds its origin in the Greek word *pharmaco*, meaning drugs or medicine.

NEW DRUGS

NEOPHARMAPHOBIA
Nee-o-fa-ma-foe-bee-ah
This fear of new medicine derives from the Greek words *pharmaco*, meaning medicine, and *neo*, meaning new.

MERCURIAL MEDICINES

HYDRAGYOPHOBIA
Hi-dra-gy-o-foe-bee-ah
Hydra and *gyro* are both Greek words meaning water and whirling, and give rise to this modern term.

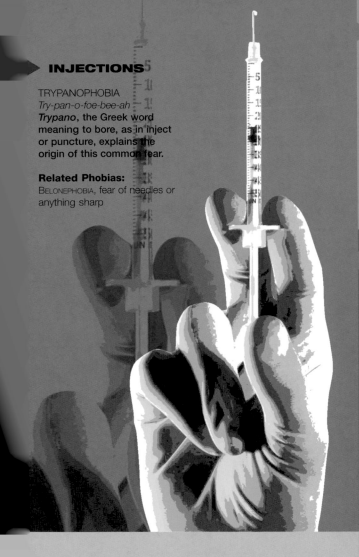

INJECTIONS

TRYPANOPHOBIA
Try-pan-o-foe-bee-ah
Trypano, the Greek word meaning to bore, as in inject or puncture, explains the origin of this common fear.

Related Phobias:
BELONEPHOBIA, fear of needles or anything sharp

VACCINATION

VACCINOPHOBIA
Vak-sin-o-foe-bee-ah
There is no Greek or Latin word that can explain the derivation of this term.

Related Phobias:
TRYPANOPHOBIA, fear of injections

DIRT, CONTAMINATION OR INFECTION

MOLYSMOPHOBIA
Mol-iss-mo-foe-bee-ah
or
MOLYSOMOPHOBIA
Mol-iss-o-mo-foe-bee-ah
or
MYSOPHOBIA
My-so-foe-bee-ah
or
MISOPHOBIA
Me-so-foe-bee-ah
Molysmophobia and molysomophobia originate from the Greek word *molysmo*, meaning infection. Mysophobia and misophopia derive in meaning from the Greek word *myso*, for filth.

Related Phobias:
MYSOPHOBIA, fear of uncleanliness
RYPOPHOBIA, fear of filth

BEING POISONED

TOXIPHOBIA
Toc-si-foe-bee-ah
or
TOXOPHOBIA
Toc-so-foe-bee-ah
or
TOXICOPHOBIA
Toc-sik-o-foe-bee-ah
Derived from the Greek word *tox*, meaning poison, this phobia also can apply to a dread of poisoning others.

HOSPITALS

NOSOCOMEPHOBIA
No-soh-ko-me-foe-bee-ah
This excessive fear of
entering a hospital in good
health and contracting an
illness while there, emanates
in meaning from the Greek
word *noso* meaning sickness.

Related Phobias:
Toxiphobia, fear of
being poisoned

DENTAL SURGERY

ODONTOPHOBIA
O-don-toe-foe-bee-ah
This fear of teeth, usually
relating to those of animals,
takes its meaning from the
Greek word *odonto*, meaning
of the tooth.

BEING AROUND DENTISTS

DENTOPHOBIA,
Den-toe-foe-bee-ah
Odonto is Greek and means of
the tooth – the Latin word for
tooth is *dent* and provides us
with contemporary words such
as dentistry and dentist.

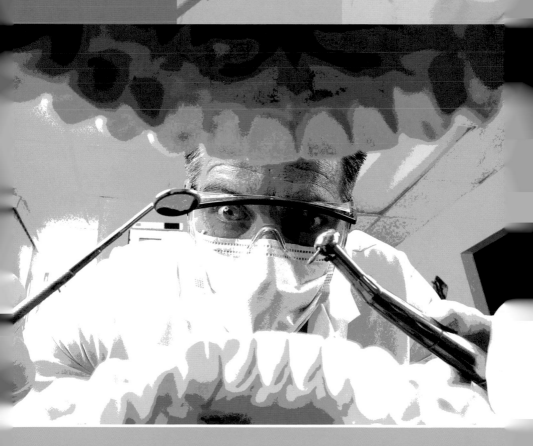

medical terms

SURGICAL OPERATION

TOMOPHOBIA
Tom-o-foe-bee-ah
This common fear emanates in meaning from the Greek suffix *tom-* meaning cut or incision.

Related Phobias:
DYSMORPHOPHOBIA, fear of deformity

SURGEONS FEAR OF OPERATING, WORK OR FUNCTIONING

ERGASIOPHOBIA
Ur-ga-si-o-foe-bee-ah
This fear derives from the Greek word *ergo*, meaning work.

Related Phobias:
XENIAPHOBIA, fear of foreign doctors

AMNESIA

AMNESIPHOBIA
Am-nee-si-foe-bee-ah
Mne, the Greek word for memory, provides us with not only the root of this term but also words like amnesty and mnemonic.

Related Phobias:
MNEMOPHOBIA, fear of memories.

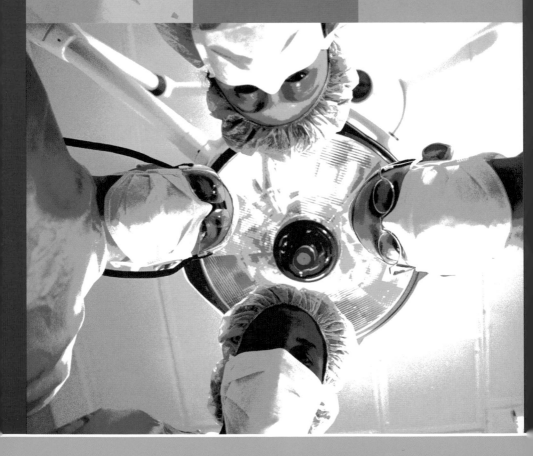

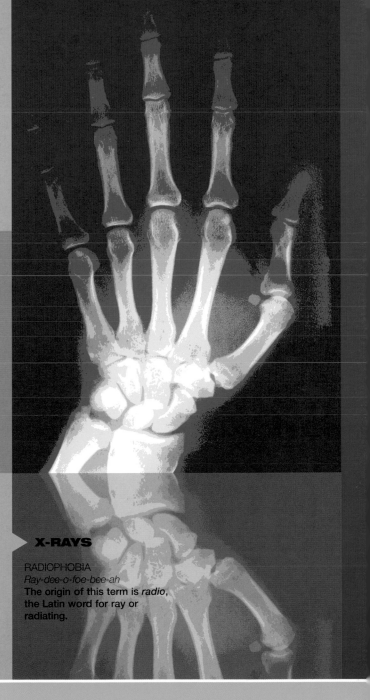

PELLAGRA

PELLAGRAPHOBIA
Pel-ag-ra-foe-bee-ah
This fear of catching pellagra, which can involve depression, irritability, and dermatitis, stems from the Greek suffix *-agra*, which means prey or seizure.

Related Phobias:
TAENIOPHOBIA, fear of tapeworms

INSANITY

DEMENTOPHOBIA
De-men-toe-foe-bee-ah
or
MANIAPHOBIA
May-nee-ah-foe-bee-ah
Demento is the Latin word for insanity, while *mania* is the Greek equivalent for mental chaos, which explains the origins of these phobias – both of which focus on a fear of going mad.

DEALING WITH INSANITY

LYSSOPHOBIA
Liss-o-foe-bee-ah
Lysso is the Greek word for madness or fury, illuminating the origins of this fear of having to deal with madness, either personally or someone else's.

X-RAYS

RADIOPHOBIA
Ray-dee-o-foe-bee-ah
The origin of this term is *radio*, the Latin word for ray or radiating.

medical terms **121**

SYMMETRY

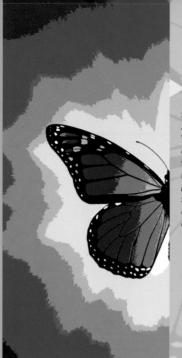

SYMMETROPHOBIA
Sim-met-row-foe-bee-ah
The origin of this fear of exactly equal things can be found in the Greek words *syn*, meaning the same, and *meter*, meaning measure. Sufferers will often rearrange ordered furniture before they can sit down.

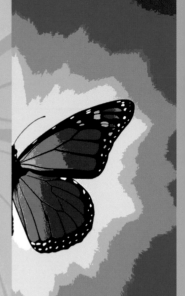

FRIDAY THE 13TH

PARASKAVEDEKATRIAPHOBIA
Para-ska-ved-ek-eh-kat-ri-a-foe-bee-ah
Para is the Greek word for wrong. Combine this the words *tri* and *deca*, meaning three and ten and we arrive at the word origin of this most commonplace fear.

Related Phobias:
MYTHOPHOBIA, fear of myths or stories incorrectly told

POINTED OBJECTS

AICHMOPHOBIA
Aye-ch-mo-foe-bee-ah
Commonly associated with a fear of needles, this phobia can be traced in origin to the Greek word *aichmo*, meaning spear.

Related Phobias:
TRYPANOPHOBIA, fear of injections

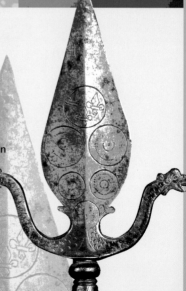

NUMBER 13

TRISKADEKAPHOBIA
Tris-ka-dek-ah-foe-bee-ah
Tri and *deca* are the Greek
words for these numbers,
which clarifies the origin of this
age-old fear of the number 13.

NUMBER 8

OCTOPHOBIA
Ok-toe-foe-bee-ah
The fear of the number eight
derives in meaning from the
Greek word for the number
eight – *octa*. From this we also
get octopus and octagon.

INFINITY

APEIROPHOBIA
A-pay-row-foe-bee-ah
Apeiro, the Greek word for
infinity or endless, gives us the
root of this anxiety.

Related Phobias:
SPACEPHOBIA, fear of outer space

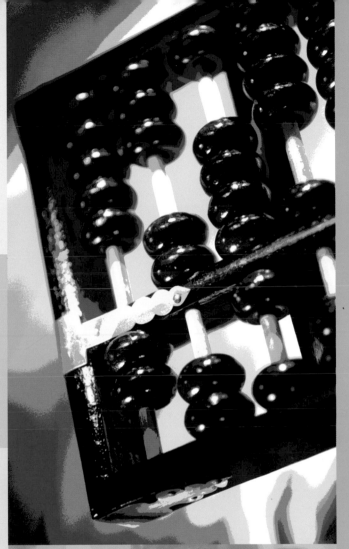

NUMBERS

ARITHMOPHOBIA
Ah-rith-mo-foe-bee-ah
or
NUMEROPHOBIA
Nu-mer-oh-foe-bee-ah

While the Greek word *arithmo*,
meaning number, provides us
with the origin of this term,
the Latin equivalent stems
from the Roman word *numer*,
meaning the same.

SYMBOLISM

SYMBOLOPHOBIA
Sim-bol-o-foe-bee-ah
There are no Greek or Latin words that can explain the origins of this term.

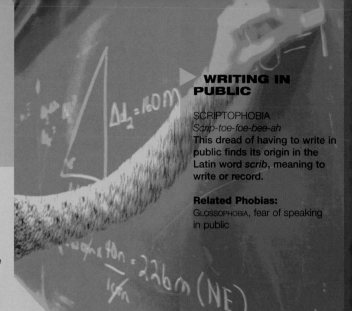

POETRY

METROPHOBIA
Met-row-foe-bee-ah
This fear of poetry derives, somewhat obscurely, from the Greek word *metro*, meaning mother or womb.

WRITING IN PUBLIC

SCRIPTOPHOBIA
Scrip-toe-foe-bee-ah
This dread of having to write in public finds its origin in the Latin word *scrib*, meaning to write or record.

Related Phobias:
GLOSSOPHOBIA, fear of speaking in public

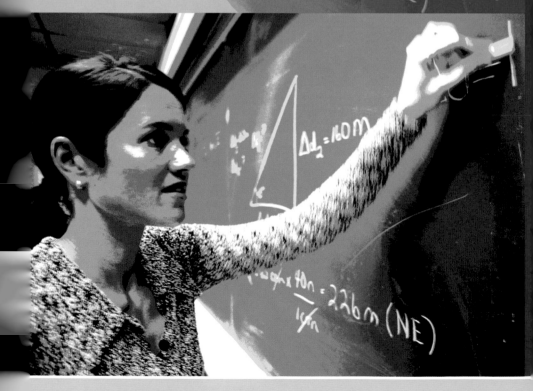

language & writing

WORDS

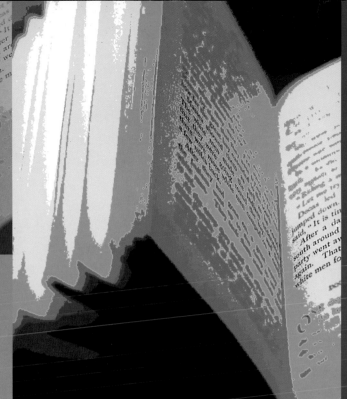

LOGOPHOBIA
Low-go-foe-bee-ah

VERBOPHOBIA
Ver-boy-foe-bee-ah
The first of these two phobias generally refers to speaking and finds its origin in the Greek verb *logo*, meaning to speak. The latter is commonly associated with a fear of words as it finds its root in the Latin word for word – *verbo*.

NAMES

NOMATOPHOBIA
Nom-at-o-foe-bee-ah
Nomen, the Latin word for name, gives us the origin of this fear.

HANDWRITING

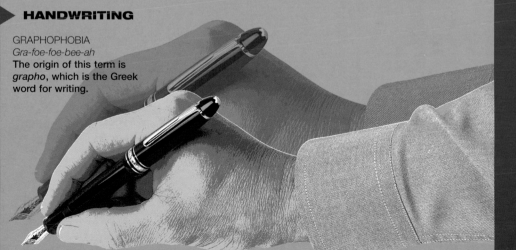

GRAPHOPHOBIA
Gra-foe-foe-bee-ah
The origin of this term is *grapho*, which is the Greek word for writing.

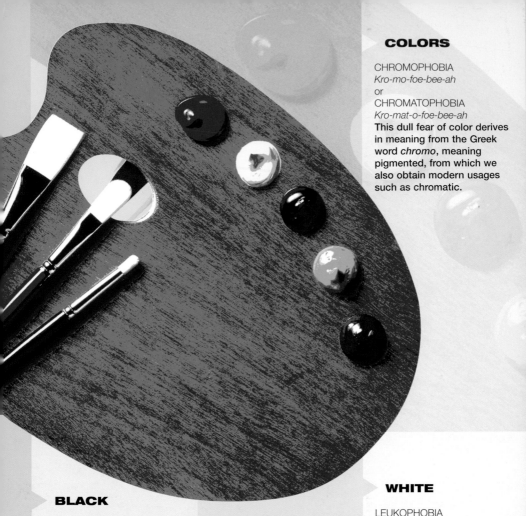

COLORS

CHROMOPHOBIA
Kro-mo-foe-bee-ah
or
CHROMATOPHOBIA
Kro-mat-o-foe-bee-ah
This dull fear of color derives in meaning from the Greek word *chromo*, **meaning pigmented, from which we also obtain modern usages such as chromatic.**

BLACK

MELANOPHOBIA
Mel-an-o-foe-bee-ah
Melano, the Greek word for black or dark, gives us the origin of this word.

Related Phobias:
NECTOPHOBIA, fear of the night

YELLOW

XANTHOPHOBIA
Zan-tho-foe-bee-ah
This particular fear can be traced in meaning to the Greek word *xantho*, meaning blonde or yellow.

WHITE

LEUKOPHOBIA
Lew-koe-foe-bee-ah
Leuko, the Greek word meaning white, gives rise to other such commonly used terms as leukemia.

Related Phobias:
PHASMOPHOBIA, fear of ghosts

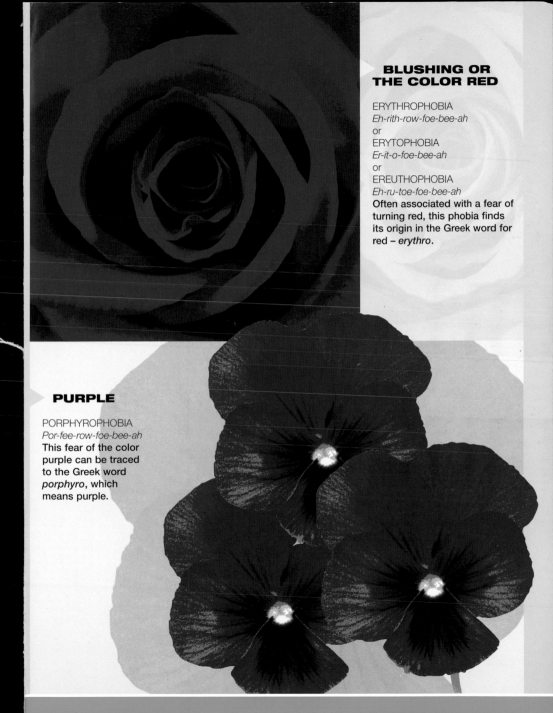

BLUSHING OR THE COLOR RED

ERYTHROPHOBIA
Eh-rith-row-foe-bee-ah
or
ERYTOPHOBIA
Er-it-o-foe-bee-ah
or
EREUTHOPHOBIA
Eh-ru-toe-foe-bee-ah
Often associated with a fear of turning red, this phobia finds its origin in the Greek word for red – *erythro*.

PURPLE

PORPHYROPHOBIA
Por-fee-row-foe-bee-ah
This fear of the color purple can be traced to the Greek word *porphyro*, which means purple.

credits

8 b NASA; 9 t NASA; 9 b U.S National Oceanic and

Atmospheric Administration; 10 tl U.S. Fish and Wildlife

Service; 10 b U.S. National Oceanic and Atmospheric

Administration; 13 r U.S. Fish and Wildlife Service;

16 tl U.S. Fish and Wildlife Service; 16 bl U.S. Fish and

Wildlife Service; 17 t U.S Fish and Wildlife Service;

17 b U.S. Fish and Wildlife Service; 18 t U.S. Fish and

Wildlife Service; 21 Corbis; 26 Corbis; 34 Colin

Anderson/Corbis; 35 Corbis; 36 Corbis; 43 Corbis;

49 t Corbis; 50 b Corbis; 54 Corbis; 55 Corbis;

59 Corbis; 61 Corbis; 64 r James W. Porter/Corbis;

64 l Image 100/Corbis 66 t Corbis; 66 br Corbis;

67 Corbis; 71 Corbis; 72 Corbis; 74 Corbis; 75 bl Corbis;

77 Corbis; 79 Corbis; 80 Corbis; 81 Corbis; 85 Corbis;

86 Image 100/Corbis; 87 Corbis; 88 Corbis; 89 Corbis;

91 Corbis; 92 Corbis; 93 Corbis; 94 t Corbis; 94 b Corbis;

99 Corbis; 101 Corbis; 102 Corbis; 103 Corbis; 104 Corbis;

105 Corbis; 106 Corbis; 107 Corbis; 108 Corbis;

109 Corbis; 110 Corbis; 112 Corbis; 115 Corbis;

117 Corbis; 118 Image 100/Corbis; 119 Corbis;

120 Corbis; 121 ER Productions/Corbis;

122 t Image 100/Corbis; 122 br Corbis; 124 Corbis;

125 t Jeffrey Coolidge/Corbis; 126 Corbis; 127 t Corbis